Written By: Gladys Stocks
Designed By: Nalani Butler & Aaron C. Butler

ISBN 9798990853263

Printed in the United States of America

BookButler Publishing Company
Upper Marlboro, MD 20774

TheBookButler.com

BookButler Publishing Company titles may be purchased in bulk for educational, business, fundraising, or sales promotional use. For information, please email: info@thebookbutler.com

BookButler
PUBLISHING COMPANY

Embracing self-love unapologetically is paramount to living a fulfilling and authentic life. When we love ourselves without reservation or apology, we grant ourselves permission to fully embody our truth and express our genuine selves. This radical self-acceptance frees us from the shackles of societal expectations and allows us to honor our unique qualities and experiences. By embracing self-love unapologetically, we cultivate a deep sense of self-worth and confidence that permeates every aspect of our lives. We learn to prioritize our needs and desires without guilt or shame, setting boundaries that protect our well-being and allow us to show up fully in our relationships and endeavors. Ultimately, unapologetically loving ourselves empowers us to navigate life with authenticity, resilience, and joy.

Gladys Stocks

Just Love Self LLC

The Self-Love Challenge: 30 Days to a Better You
is designed to guide you through a month-long exploration
of self-love, personal growth, and inner peace.

Each day, engage in activities and reflections designed to
foster a deeper appreciation and compassion for yourself.
Remember, self-love is a journey. Every step you take
is a step towards a happier and more fulfilled life.

Turn the page to start this empowering
journey towards a better you.

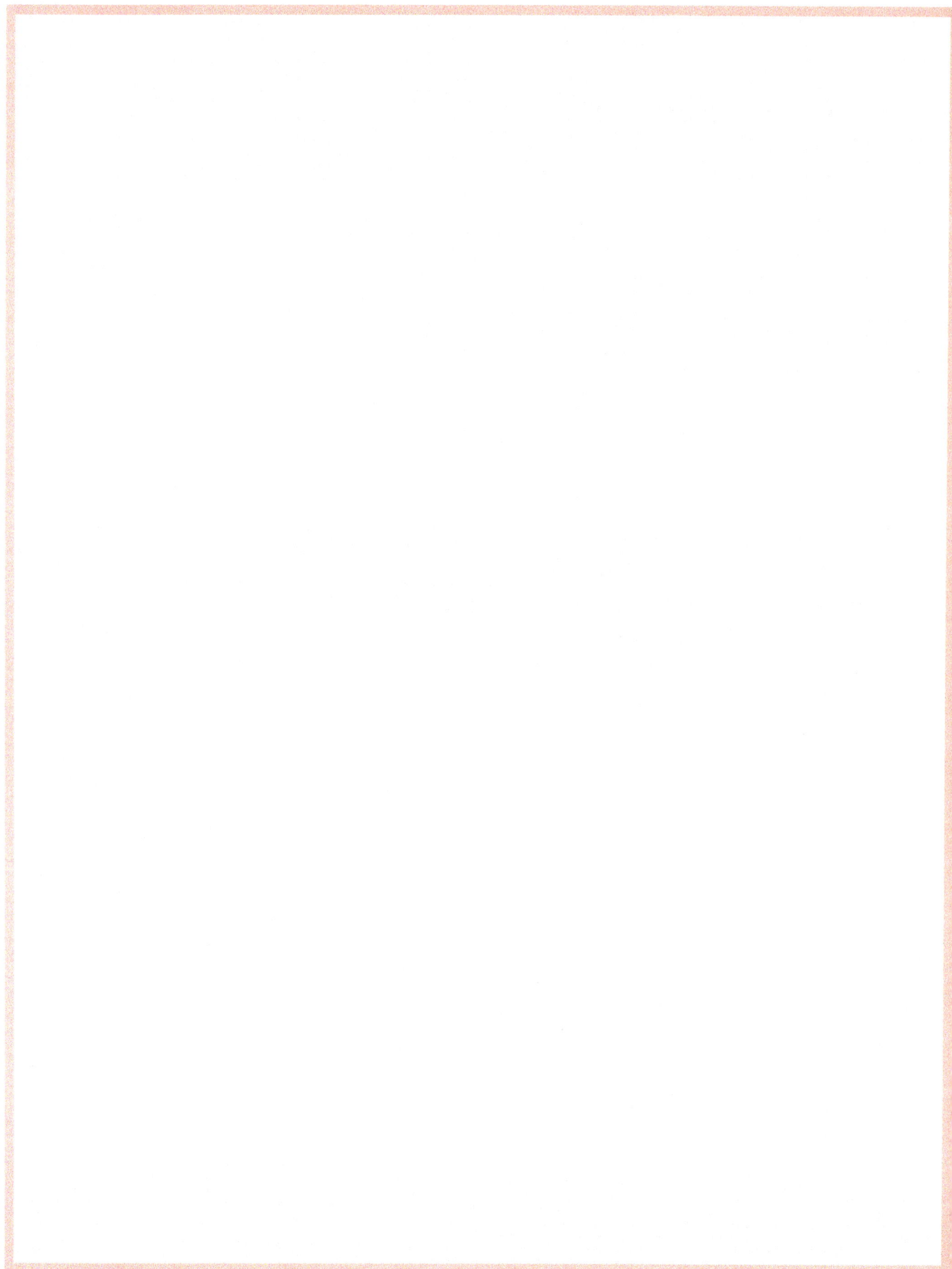

The Self-Love Challenge

DAYS 1-10 | MOTIVATION AND UNDERSTANDING SELF-CARE

Journal

Practice gratitude

Plan Self-Care

Write a letter to yourself

Self-Love Affirmations

Practice positive visualization

Set Boundaries

Do something kind for yourself

Exercise

Meditate

DAY 1: Self-Love Affirmations

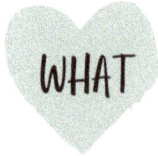

WHAT

Write down five affirmations that uplift and empower you. Repeat them to yourself throughout the day to foster a positive and loving mindset.

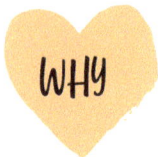

WHY

Affirmations are positive statements that can help you challenge and overcome self-sabotaging and negative thoughts. When you repeat them often and believe in them, you can start to make positive changes.

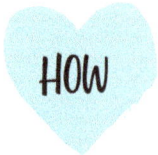

HOW

Crafting your Affirmations:
- Think positively. Focus on what you want to achieve rather than what you want to avoid.
- Use "I" statements to make the affirmations personal and allow them to resonate with you.
- Focus on specific qualities or attributes you want to embrace or enhance.

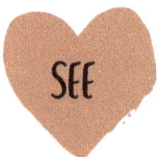

SEE

Examples of Positive Affirmations:
- "I am confident and capable."
- "I am strong, resilient, and brave."
- "I am proud of who I am and all I have accomplished."
- "I am worthy of love and respect."
- "I deserve to take care of myself and put my needs first."
- "I am enough just as I am."

GROW

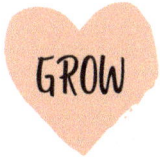

Incorporating Affirmations into Your Day.

Morning Routine:
Start your day by reading your affirmations out loud with conviction. This sets a positive tone for the day ahead.

Throughout the Day:
Whenever you notice negative self-talk or feel stressed, pause and repeat your affirmations. This helps to shift your mindset.

Evening Routine:
End your day by reflecting on your affirmations. Consider how they have influenced your thoughts and actions throughout the day.

Note: By integrating self-love affirmations into your daily routine, you start to build a habit of positive self-talk that nurtures your self-esteem and overall well-being. Enjoy this empowering start to your self-love journey!

Affirmations

1

2

3

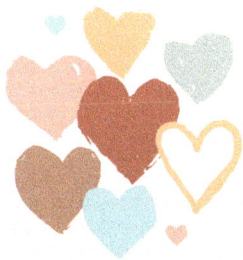

Reflective Practice

At the end of Day 1, take some time to reflect on how using affirmations made you feel. Write down any observations, such as:

- Did the affirmations help shift your mindset?
- How did you feel before and after repeating your affirmations?
- Were there any moments where the affirmations felt particularly powerful or needed?

DAY 2: Gratitude Journal

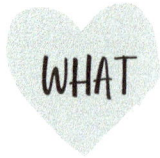

WHAT

List five things you're grateful for about yourself. Reflect on why each of these qualities or attributes is valuable to foster a deeper self-appreciation.

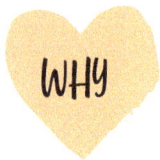

WHY

Gratitude journaling focuses on recognizing and appreciating positive aspects of yourself. This practice can enhance your mood, increase self-esteem, and promote a more positive outlook on life.

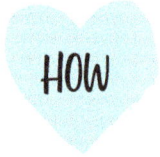

HOW

Identifying Areas of Gratitude:
Consider qualities, skills, experiences, and attributes that you appreciate about yourself. These could be aspects of your personality, achievements, physical traits, or ways you handle situations.

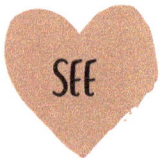

SEE

Examples of Gratitude Entries:
- **Quality**: Kindness
- **Reflection**: "I am grateful for my kindness because it allows me to connect deeply with others and make them feel valued and loved."

- **Quality**: Creativity
- **Reflection**: "I am grateful for my creativity because it brings joy and innovation to my life and the lives of others."

GROW

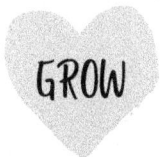

Incorporating Gratitude into Your Day.

Morning Routine:
Start your day by reading your gratitude list to remind yourself of your positive qualities.

Throughout the Day:
Take moments to reflect on your gratitude entries, especially during challenging times. Let these reflections boost your confidence and mood.

Evening Routine:
End your day by reviewing your gratitude list and adding any new qualities or attributes you discovered throughout the day.

***Note:** By integrating gratitude journaling into your daily routine, you start to build a habit of recognizing and appreciating your positive attributes, which can significantly enhance your self-love and overall well-being. Enjoy this reflective and empowering practice!*

Gratitude Journaling

QUALITY

REFLECTION

QUALITY

REFLECTION

QUALITY

REFLECTION

QUALITY

REFLECTION

QUALITY

REFLECTION

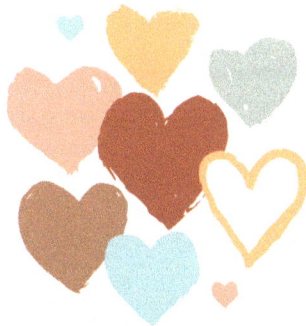

Reflective Practice

At the end of Day 2, take some time to reflect on your gratitude journaling experience. Write down any observations, such as:

- How did focusing on gratitude affect your mood and mindset?
- Did you discover any new qualities about yourself that you hadn't recognized before?
- How did acknowledging these qualities help you during the day?

DAY 3: Self-Care Plan

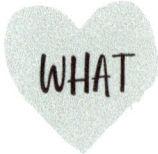

WHAT

Create a realistic and obtainable self-care plan for the week ahead. This plan should include activities that nourish your body, mind, and soul, and be tailored to fit into your current lifestyle.

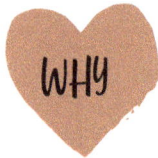

WHY

A self-care plan helps you balance your mental, physical, and emotional needs while reminding you of the important people in your support system and the self-care goals you wish to accomplish.

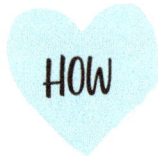

HOW

Crafting Your Self-Care Plan:
- Assess your needs for your mind, body, and soul.
  - Body: Consider what your body needs to feel healthy and energized. This can include exercise, nutrition, rest, and hygiene.
  - Mind: Think about activities that stimulate and relax your mind. This might involve hobbies, reading, learning, and mental breaks.
  - Soul: Reflect on what nurtures your inner self and brings you joy and peace. This can include spiritual practices, creative outlets, nature, and connections with loved ones.

- Identify specific goals for each area of self-care (mind, body, soul).
- Create a schedule to achieve your goals. Be realistic.

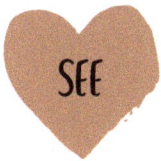

SEE

Example of a Day in a Self-Care Plan:

Monday
- Morning: 20 minutes of yoga
- Afternoon: Listen to a podcast during a commute
- Evening: 10 minutes of journaling

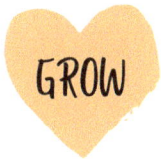

GROW

Incorporating Flexibility into Your Plan.

Be flexible and forgiving with yourself. If you miss an activity, don't be discouraged. Adjust your plan as needed and continue with a positive mindset.

Note: *By creating a realistic and obtainable self-care plan, you're setting yourself up for a week filled with activities that nourish your body, mind, and soul. Enjoy your journey and remember to be kind to yourself!*

Self-Care Plan

MORNING	AFTERNOON	EVENING
PLAN	PLAN	PLAN

NOTES

MORNING	AFTERNOON	EVENING
PLAN	PLAN	PLAN

NOTES

MORNING	AFTERNOON	EVENING
PLAN	PLAN	PLAN

NOTES

MORNING	AFTERNOON	EVENING
PLAN	PLAN	PLAN

NOTES

Day 3

MORNING	AFTERNOON	EVENING
PLAN	PLAN	PLAN

NOTES

MORNING	AFTERNOON	EVENING
PLAN	PLAN	PLAN

NOTES

MORNING	AFTERNOON	EVENING
PLAN	PLAN	PLAN

NOTES

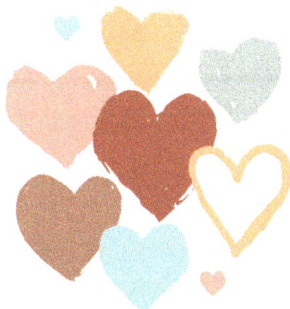

Day 3

Reflective Practice

At the end of the week, reflect on what worked and what didn't. Adjust your self-care plan based on your reflections to better fit your needs and schedule for the next week. Write down any observations.

DAY 4: Letter to Yourself

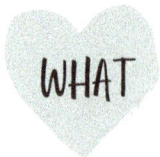

WHAT

Write a heartfelt letter to yourself, expressing love, kindness, and encouragement. Read it aloud with compassion to foster a deeper sense of self-love and appreciation.

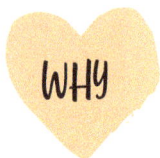

WHY

Writing a heartfelt letter to yourself is a powerful exercise in self-compassion and self-acceptance. This activity allows you to express love, kindness, and encouragement to yourself, reinforcing positive self-talk and strengthening your emotional well-being. By acknowledging your own worth and offering yourself the same compassion you would offer a dear friend, you cultivate a deeper sense of self-love and inner peace.

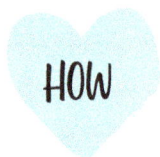

HOW

Crafting Your Letter:
- Find a quiet, comfortable space where you won't be disturbed. Consider playing soft music or lighting a candle to create a relaxing atmosphere.
- Reflect on your journey. Think about your strengths, your achievements, and the challenges you've overcome. Recognize the qualities you admire about yourself and the progress you've made.

- Write your letter.
  - Write about your positive qualities and achievements. Be specific and genuine.
  - Offer words of encouragement and support. Acknowledge any struggles and remind yourself of your resilience and capability.
  - Include affirmations and promises to continue caring for and believing in yourself.
- Read your letter aloud. Listen to your words and let them sink in. Feel the love and kindness you are giving to yourself.

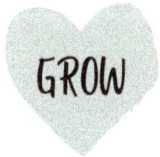

GROW

Incorporating Your Letter into Your Day.

Morning Routine:
Start your day by reading your letter to yourself. Let it set a positive and encouraging tone for the day.

Throughout the Day:
Reflect on the words of your letter whenever you need a boost of self-love and encouragement.

Evening Routine:
End your day by reading your letter once more. Allow it to soothe and comfort you as you wind down for the night.

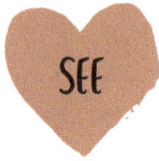

Example of a Letter:

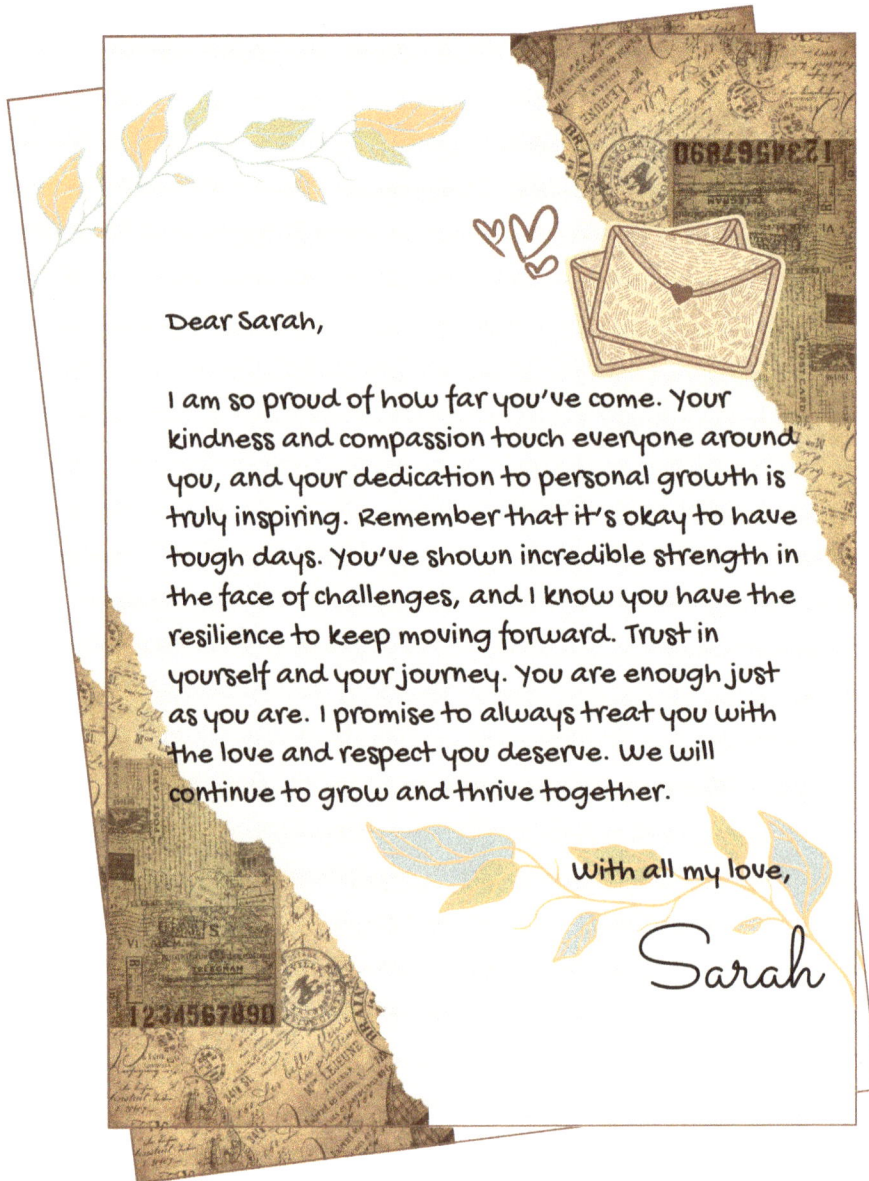

Dear Sarah,

I am so proud of how far you've come. Your kindness and compassion touch everyone around you, and your dedication to personal growth is truly inspiring. Remember that it's okay to have tough days. You've shown incredible strength in the face of challenges, and I know you have the resilience to keep moving forward. Trust in yourself and your journey. You are enough just as you are. I promise to always treat you with the love and respect you deserve. We will continue to grow and thrive together.

With all my love,

Sarah

Note: *By writing a heartfelt letter to yourself and incorporating it into your daily routine, you are actively nurturing your self-love and fostering a deeper connection with yourself. Enjoy this meaningful and empowering practice!*

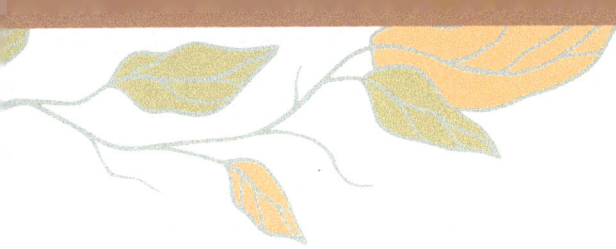
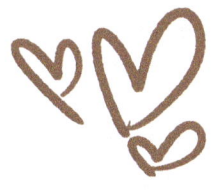
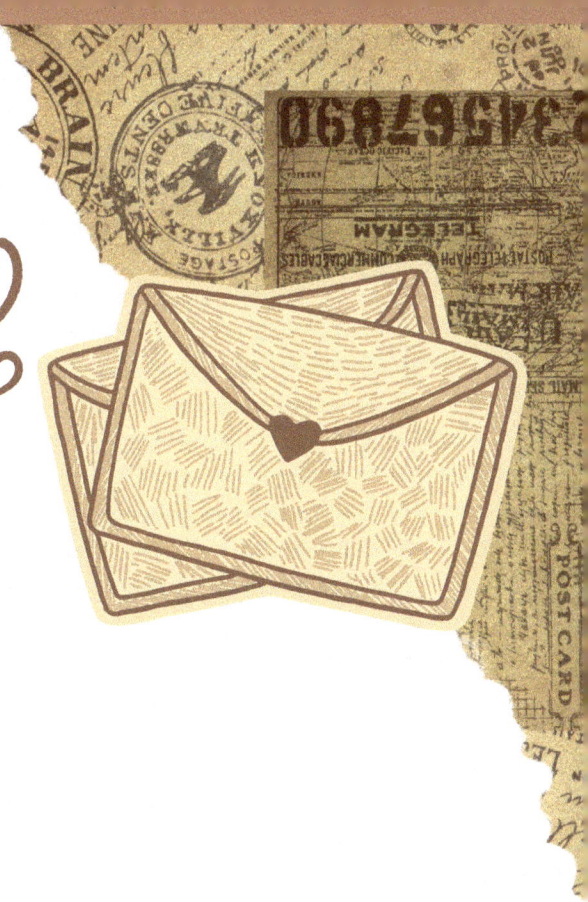
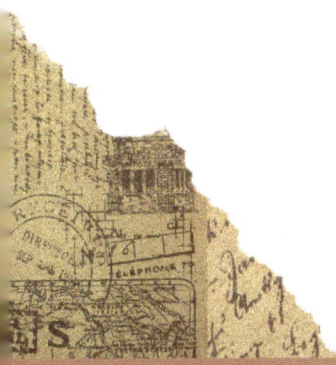
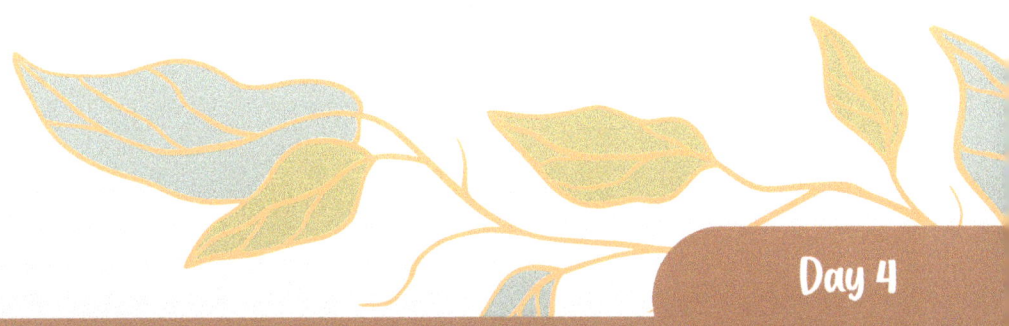

Day 4

Reflective Practice

At the end of Day 4, take some time to reflect on how writing and reading your letter affected you. Write down any observations, such as:

- How did expressing love and kindness to yourself make you feel?
- Did reading the letter aloud help reinforce the positive messages?
- How did the letter influence your thoughts and emotions throughout the day?

DAY 5: Mindfulness Meditation

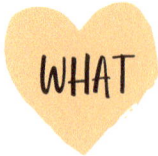

WHAT
Practice a guided mindfulness meditation focusing on self-compassion and acceptance. This practice helps you cultivate a deeper sense of self-awareness and kindness towards yourself.

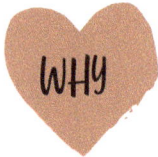

WHY
Mindfulness meditation involves paying attention to the present moment without judgment. It helps reduce stress, improve focus, and increase self-compassion and acceptance.

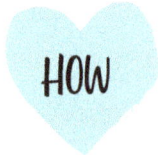

HOW
Getting Ready for Meditation:
- Find a quiet, comfortable place where you won't be disturbed. Sit in a comfortable position, either on a chair or on the floor with a cushion. Ensure your back is straight but relaxed.
- Search for mindfulness meditation videos on YouTube that focus on self-compassion and acceptance. Choose the video you feel will work best for you.
- Take a few deep breaths to center yourself and prepare your mind for meditation. Aim for 10-20 minutes.

SEE

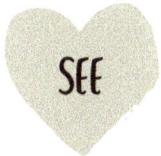

Play the chosen guided meditation video and follow the prompts. Focus on the words and let them guide your thoughts and feelings.

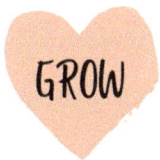

GROW

Incorporating Mindfulness into Your Day.

Morning Routine:
Start your day with a short 5-minute mindfulness meditation to set a calm and focused tone.

Throughout the Day:
Practice mindful breathing during breaks or stressful moments. Focus on your breathing for a few minutes to re-center yourself.

Evening Routine:
End your day with a longer mindfulness meditation session to unwind and reflect on your day with compassion.

Note: *By incorporating mindfulness meditation into your daily routine, you are cultivating a practice that promotes self-compassion, acceptance, and overall well-being. Enjoy the calming and centering benefits of this meaningful practice!*

Mindfulness Meditation

CLICK FOR VIDEO OPTIONS

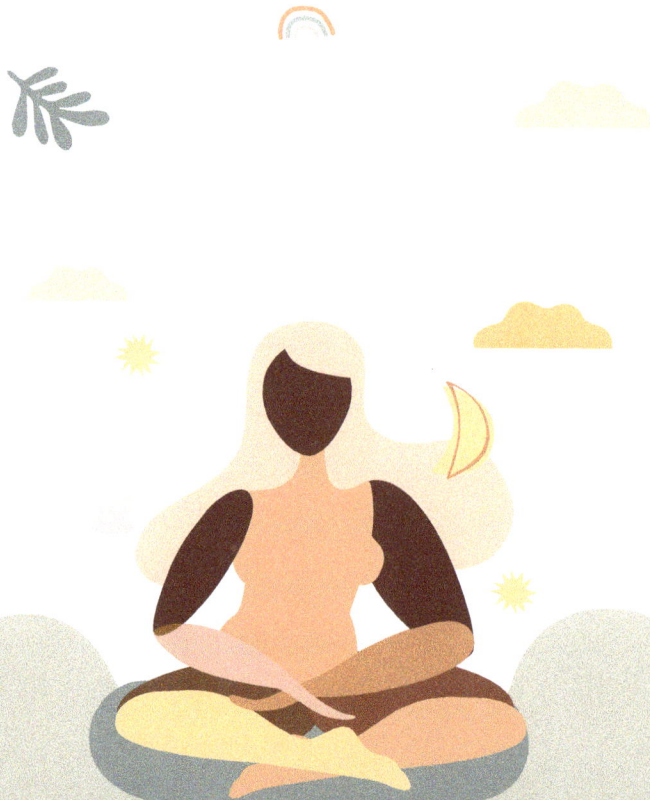

Self-Guided Meditation

**If you prefer a self-guided practice,
follow these steps:**

Close your eyes and take a few deep breaths, inhaling deeply through
your nose and exhaling slowly through your mouth.

Bring your attention to your breathing. Notice the sensation
of the air entering and leaving your body.

As thoughts arise, acknowledge them without judgment and gently
bring your focus back to your breath.

Gradually shift your focus to self-compassion and acceptance. Repeat
phrases like, "May I be kind to myself," "May I accept myself as I am,"
and "May I be at peace."

Visualize yourself surrounded by a warm, loving light. Allow it to
fill you with feelings of compassion and acceptance.

Reflective Practice

At the end of Day 5, take some time to reflect on your mindfulness meditation experience. Write down any observations, such as:

- How did practicing mindfulness meditation make you feel?
- Did you notice any changes in your stress levels or emotional state?
- How did focusing on self-compassion and acceptance influence your thoughts and feelings about yourself?

DAY 6: Positive Visualization

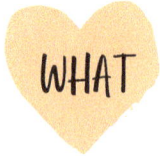

WHAT

Visualize yourself succeeding and feeling confident in a challenging situation. Hold on to this image throughout the day to build confidence and a positive mindset.

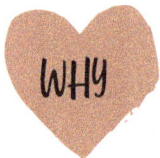

WHY

Positive visualization involves creating a mental image of yourself achieving your goals and confidently handling challenging situations. This technique can boost your self-esteem and motivation by helping you mentally rehearse success.

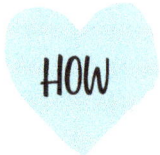

HOW

Getting Ready for Visualization:
- Think of a specific situation where you want to feel more confident and succeed. This could be a work presentation, a difficult conversation, a personal goal, or any scenario that challenges you.
- Find a quiet, comfortable space where you won't be disturbed. Sit or lie down in a relaxed position, close your eyes, and take a few deep breaths to center yourself.

SEE

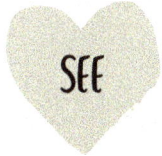

Practicing Positive Visualization:
- Close Your Eyes and Relax:
  - Take a few deep breaths, inhaling through your nose and exhaling through your mouth. Let go of any tension in your body.
- Create a Clear Mental Image:
  - Picture the challenging situation in your mind. Visualize yourself in the setting where the event will take place.
- Visualize Success:
  - See yourself handling the situation with confidence and ease. Imagine speaking clearly, making positive decisions, or performing the task successfully.
- Engage All Senses:
  - Include as much detail as possible. Imagine the sounds, smells, and sensations associated with the situation. Feel the emotions of confidence, success, and satisfaction.
- Hold On to the Positive Image:
  - Focus on this positive image and the feelings of success and confidence. Allow these feelings to fill you with a sense of empowerment and readiness.

GROW

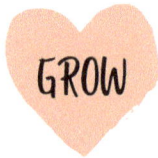

Incorporating Visualization into Your Day.

Morning Routine:
Start your day with a 5 to 10-minute positive visualization session to set a confident tone.

Throughout the Day:
Whenever you feel doubt or anxiety, take a moment to recall your visualization. Remind yourself of the confident and successful image.

Evening Routine:
End your day by reflecting on your visualization experience and reinforcing the positive image for future reference.

Note: *By incorporating positive visualization into your daily routine, you are training your mind to focus on success and confidence, which can significantly enhance your overall well-being and performance. Enjoy the empowering and uplifting benefits of this practice!*

Visualize & Draw

Reflective Practice

At the end of Day 6, take some time to reflect on your positive visualization experience. Write down any observations, such as:

- How did the visualization make you feel before and during the challenging situation?
- Did you notice any changes in your confidence levels or emotional state?
- How did holding onto the positive image influence your actions and mindset throughout the day?

DAY 7: Acts of Self-Kindness

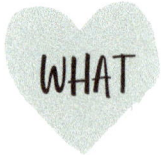

WHAT
Perform a random act of kindness for yourself to show self-love and care. This act can be as simple as treating yourself to a favorite meal or indulging in a hobby you love.

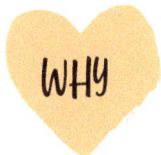

WHY
Acts of kindness towards yourself are essential for self-love and well-being. They reinforce the idea that you deserve care and appreciation, and they can boost your mood and reduce stress.

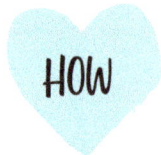

HOW
Crafting your Acts of Kindness:
- Think about activities or treats that make you happy and relaxed
- Choose an act of kindness that you can realistically fit into your day.
- Set aside time to fully enjoy and engage in this act without rushing or feeling guilty.

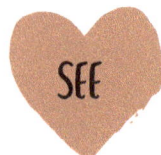

SEE
Examples of Acts of Kindness:
- Treat yourself to a favorite meal
- Indulge in a hobby
- Relax with a spa day at home
- Take a nature walk
- Buy yourself a small gift

GROW

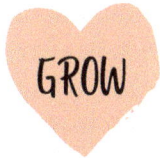

Incorporating Acts of Self-Kindness into Your Day.

Morning Routine:
Start your day by planning your act of kindness. Think about what would bring you joy and relaxation today.

Throughout the Day:
Perform your act of kindness. Tip: You don't need to stop there. Find other moments to treat yourself throughout the day!

Evening Routine:
End your day by reflecting on your act(s) of kindness. Think about how doing these activities for yourself made you feel.

Note: By incorporating acts of kindness into your daily routine, you are actively nurturing your self-love and reinforcing the idea that you deserve care and appreciation. Enjoy the positive and uplifting effects of this practice!

Ideas for Acts of Self-Kindness

Reflective Practice

At the end of Day 7, take some time to reflect on your acts of kindness experience. Write down any observations, such as:

- How did performing acts of kindness for yourself make you feel?
- Did you notice any changes in your mood or stress levels?
- How did taking time for yourself impact your overall well-being?

Day 7

DAY 8: Reflective Journaling

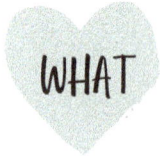

WHAT

Reflect on a time when you felt proud of yourself. Write about the experience and acknowledge your strengths and achievements. This practice helps reinforce positive self-recognition and appreciation.

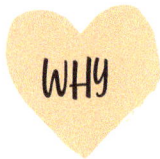

WHY

Reflective journaling helps you connect with your past experiences and recognize your accomplishments. It reinforces positive self-perception and highlights your strengths, boosting your self-esteem.

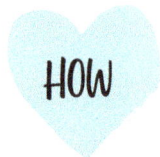

HOW

Writing Your Journal Entry:
- Recall a moment when you felt proud of yourself.
- Describe the situation, your actions, and the outcome.
- Acknowledge personal strengths and qualities that helped you achieve this proud moment.
- Reflect on what you learned from the experience.

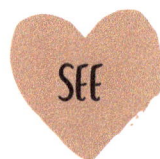

SEE

Example of Reflective Journaling:
- Recall: "I remember the day I gave my first public speech at a community event. I had prepared for weeks and was both excited and nervous."

- Describe: "Standing at the podium, I could see the supportive faces in the audience. I took a deep breath and began my speech. As I spoke, I felt more confident with each word. The audience was engaged, and I received applause and positive feedback afterward."
- Acknowledge: "My determination, preparation, and ability to stay calm under pressure helped me succeed. I realized I could communicate effectively and inspire others."
- Reflect: "This experience boosted my confidence and motivated me to take on more public speaking opportunities. It reminded me of my potential to overcome fears and achieve my goals.

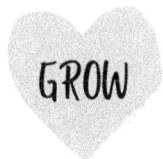

GROW

Incorporating Constructive Feedback into Your Reflective Journaling.

Identify potential areas for improvement in your experience. By recognizing the room you still have to grow, you can strive towards becoming a better you.

Note: *By incorporating reflective journaling into your daily routine, you are actively nurturing self-recognition and appreciation, which can significantly enhance your self-esteem and personal growth. Enjoy the empowering and affirming effects of this practice!*

Reflective Journaling Prompt

Morning Activity: Start your day by thinking about a moment when you felt proud of yourself. Reflect on the details and emotions associated with that experience.
- **Example Reflection:** Recall the day you received a promotion at work due to your hard work and dedication.

Midday Activity: During a break, jot down any additional thoughts or details about the experience that come to mind.
- **Example Note:** Remember how your colleagues congratulated you and how validated and appreciated you felt.

Evening Activity: In the evening, dedicate time to write a detailed account of your proud moment.
- **Example Entry:**
  - **Recall the Experience:** I remember the day I was promoted to a leadership position at work. It was a culmination of years of hard work and dedication.
  - **Describe the Experience:** My manager called me into their office and shared the good news. I felt a rush of pride and excitement. My colleagues congratulated me, and I felt truly valued.
  - **Acknowledge Your Strengths:** My commitment, leadership skills, and ability to collaborate effectively were key to my promotion. I realized my potential to lead and inspire others.
  - **Reflect on the Impact:** This promotion boosted my confidence and motivated me to continue growing professionally. It reinforced my belief in my abilities and dedication.

Reflective Practice

At the end of Day 8, take some time to reflect on your journaling experience. Write down any observations, such as:

- How did reflecting on a proud moment make you feel?
- Did you notice any changes in your self-perception or mood?
- How did acknowledging your strengths and achievements influence your overall well-being?

DAY 9: Setting Boundaries

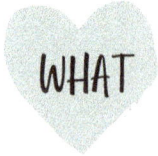

WHAT

Identify one boundary you need to establish to honor your well-being. Communicate it assertively and kindly to protect your mental and emotional health.

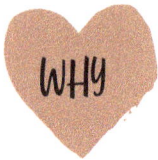

WHY

Boundaries are essential for maintaining healthy relationships and protecting your mental and emotional well-being. They help you define what is acceptable and unacceptable behavior from others.

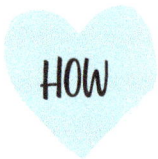

HOW

Establishing Effective Boundaries:
- Identify the Boundary: Reflect on areas in your life where you feel overwhelmed, disrespected, or stressed. Select one that is important to your well-being. Be specific about what you need and why it is necessary.
- Communicate the Boundary Assertively and Kindly: Plan how you will communicate your boundary. Be clear, direct, and kind. Use "I" statements to express your needs without blaming or criticizing others.
- Follow Through and Maintain the Boundary: Consistently enforce the boundary you set. Be prepared to remind others of your boundary if necessary and stay firm in your decision.

SEE

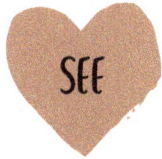

Example of Setting and Communicating a Boundary:

- Boundary at Work: Limiting work-related communication after office hours to maintain work-life balance.
- Communicate the Boundary: "I value our team's communication, but I need to maintain a work-life balance. Starting this week, I won't be checking work emails after 7 PM. If something is urgent, please call me directly."

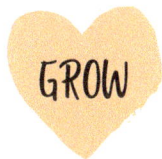

GROW

Incorporating Boundaries for Healthier Relationships

Without boundaries, relationships deteriorate, leading to overwhelm and resentment. Be realistic about situations at work, with family, and friends, or in other relationships where clear boundaries are necessary.

Note: *By incorporating boundary-setting into your daily routine, you are actively taking steps to protect your well-being and enhance your relationships. Enjoy the empowering and liberating effects of this practice!*

Reflective Practice

At the end of Day 9, take some time to reflect on your boundary-setting experience. Write down any observations, such as:

- How did identifying and setting a boundary make you feel?
- Were you able to communicate your boundary assertively and kindly?
- How did others react to your boundary? How did their reactions make you feel?
- How do you plan to maintain this boundary moving forward?

DAY 10: Self-Compassion

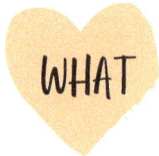

WHAT

Practice self-compassion by treating yourself as you would a dear friend facing a similar struggle. This exercise helps you develop kindness and understanding towards yourself, especially during challenging times.

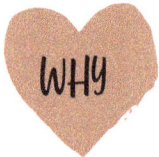

WHY

Self-compassion involves being kind and understanding towards yourself, especially when you are experiencing difficulties or self-doubt. It helps reduce negative self-talk and promotes emotional resilience.

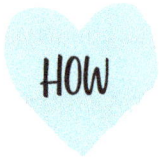

HOW

Practicing Self-Compassion:
- Think about a challenge or difficulty you are currently facing. This could be in any area where you feel stressed or inadequate.
- Imagine a friend facing the same struggle and think about how you would respond to them, what you would say, and how you would offer support and encouragement.
- Write a letter to yourself, addressing yourself with kindness, understanding, and encouragement.
- Read the letter aloud and allow the words to uplift you.
- Take a moment to reflect on how this experience made you feel.

SEE

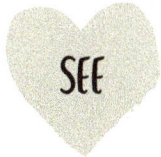

- Example of the Structure for the Letter:
  - Greeting: Begin with a warm and caring greeting, such as "Dear [Your Name]," or "My dear friend,"
  - Acknowledge the Struggle: Acknowledge the difficulty you are facing with empathy. For example, "I know you are going through a tough time right now, and it's okay to feel overwhelmed."
  - Offer Support and Encouragement: Provide words of support and encouragement, just as you would to a friend. For example, "You are strong and capable. Remember all the times you have overcome challenges before."
  - Remind Yourself of Your Worth: Reinforce your self-worth and remind yourself of your strengths. For example, "You deserve love and kindness, especially from yourself. You are doing the best you can, and that is enough."
  - Closing: End with a positive and caring closing, such as "With love and compassion," or "Always here for you,"

GROW

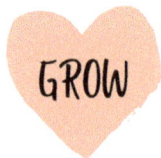

Incorporating Self-Compassion into Your Daily Practice.

Recognize the importance of treating yourself with the same kindness and understanding that you would offer a friend. By acknowledging your struggles and encouraging yourself, you can build emotional resilience and foster a deeper sense of self-worth.

Note: *By incorporating self-compassion into your daily routine, you are nurturing a kinder and more supportive relationship with yourself. Enjoy the comforting and healing effects of this practice!*

Practice Self-Compassion

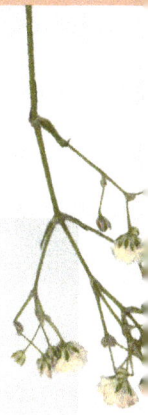

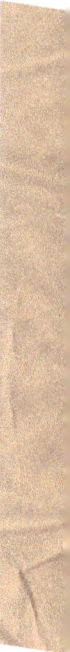
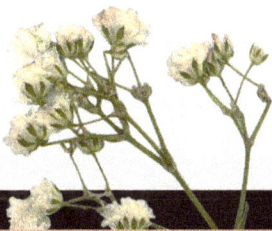
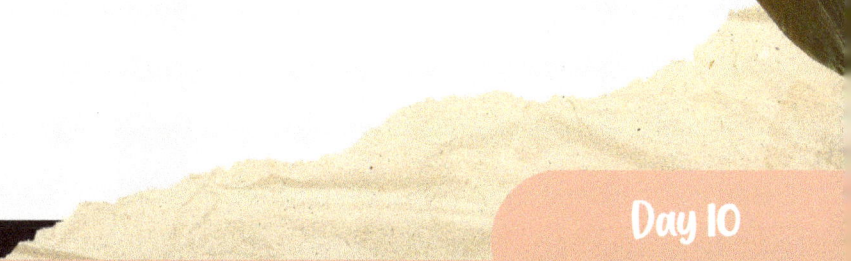

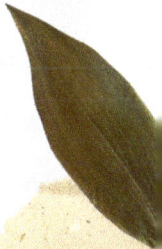

Reflective Practice

At the end of Day 10, take some time to reflect on your self-compassion exercise. Write down any observations, such as:

- How did practicing self-compassion make you feel?
- Did you notice any changes in your self-talk or emotional state?
- How did treating yourself with the same kindness you would offer a friend impact your overall well-being?

The Self-Love Challenge

Affirm

Create a
self-love playlist

Avoid
social media

Challenge
negative
thoughts

Body
Appreciation

Self Discovery
Assessment

Create a personal
growth plan

Do something
creative

Nature

Support

DAY 11: Affectionate Self-Talk

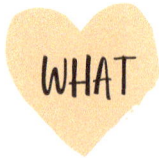

WHAT
Replace self-criticism with gentle, loving self-talk. Challenge negative thoughts with affirmations of self-worth to promote a positive and nurturing inner dialogue.

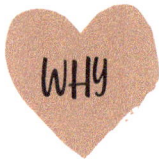

WHY
Self-talk is your inner dialogue. Affectionate self-talk means speaking to yourself with kindness, understanding, and encouragement, which can boost your self-esteem and emotional well-being.

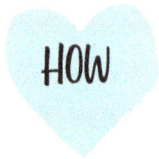

HOW
Using Affectionate Self-Talk:
- Identify Self-Critical Thoughts
- Challenge Negative Thoughts
- Replace with Gentle, Loving Self-Talk
- Practice Affectionate Self-Talk Throughout the day
- Reflect on the Experience

*Tip: Create a list of affirmations that resonate with you. Keep this list handy to refer to when you need.

SEE

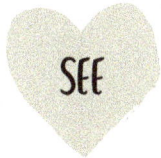

Examples of Affirmations:
- "I trust myself to make the right decisions."
- "I am proud of my progress and achievements."
- "I am enough just as I am."

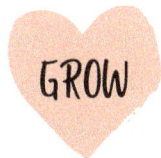

GROW

Incorporating Affectionate Self-Talk into Your Day.

Morning Routine:
Identify common self-critical thoughts. Commit to challenging and replacing them with positive affirmations.

Throughout the Day:
Pay attention to your inner dialogue. When you notice negative thoughts, pause and replace them with affirmations.

Evening Routine:
Reflect on your day and how practicing affectionate self-talk impacted you. Write down any observations or feelings.

Note: *By incorporating affectionate self-talk into your daily routine, you are fostering a more positive and supportive inner dialogue. Enjoy the uplifting and empowering effects of this practice!*

Self-Talk Reflective Art

Objective: Creativity and reflection while practicing affectionate self-talk.

Transform a Thought: In the bubble below, write a negative self-critical thought you commonly have. On the opposite page in the thought bubble, rewrite the negative thought as a positive affirmation using affectionate self-talk. Use colorful pens or markers to make it stand out.
- Negative Thought Example: "I always mess things up."
- Transformed Affirmation: "I am learning and growing with each experience. It's okay to make mistakes."

Decorate the Bubble: Decorate the positive thought bubble with drawings and patterns that make it visually appealing and uplifting. This can include hearts, stars, flowers, or any symbols that represent positivity to you.

Illustrate Your Day: Around the bubbles, draw or doodle small scenes or icons that represent moments from your day when you practiced affectionate self-talk. For example, you might draw a sun or a coffee cup to represent your morning routine, a briefcase or computer for work tasks, or a moon or book for your evening reflection.

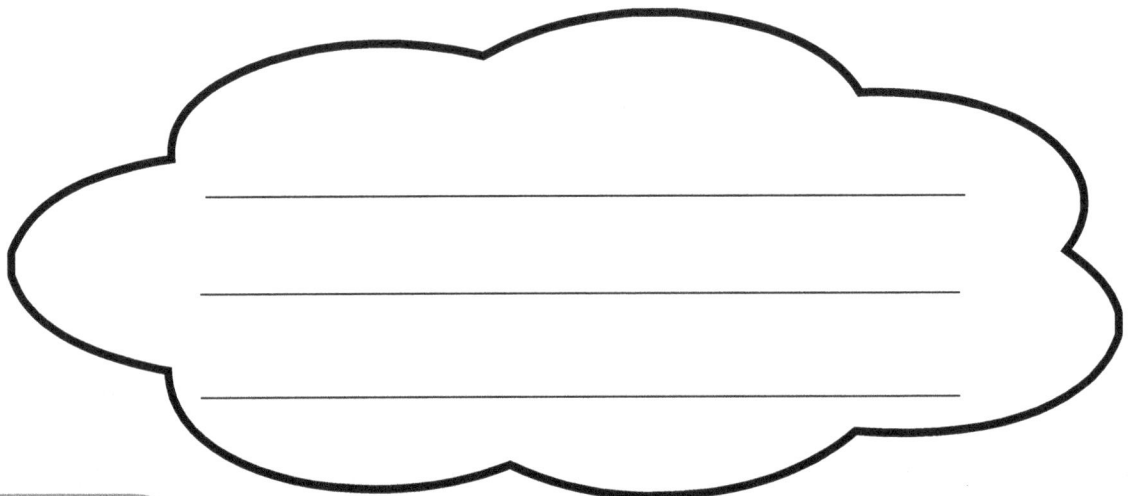

_____

_____

_____

Day 11

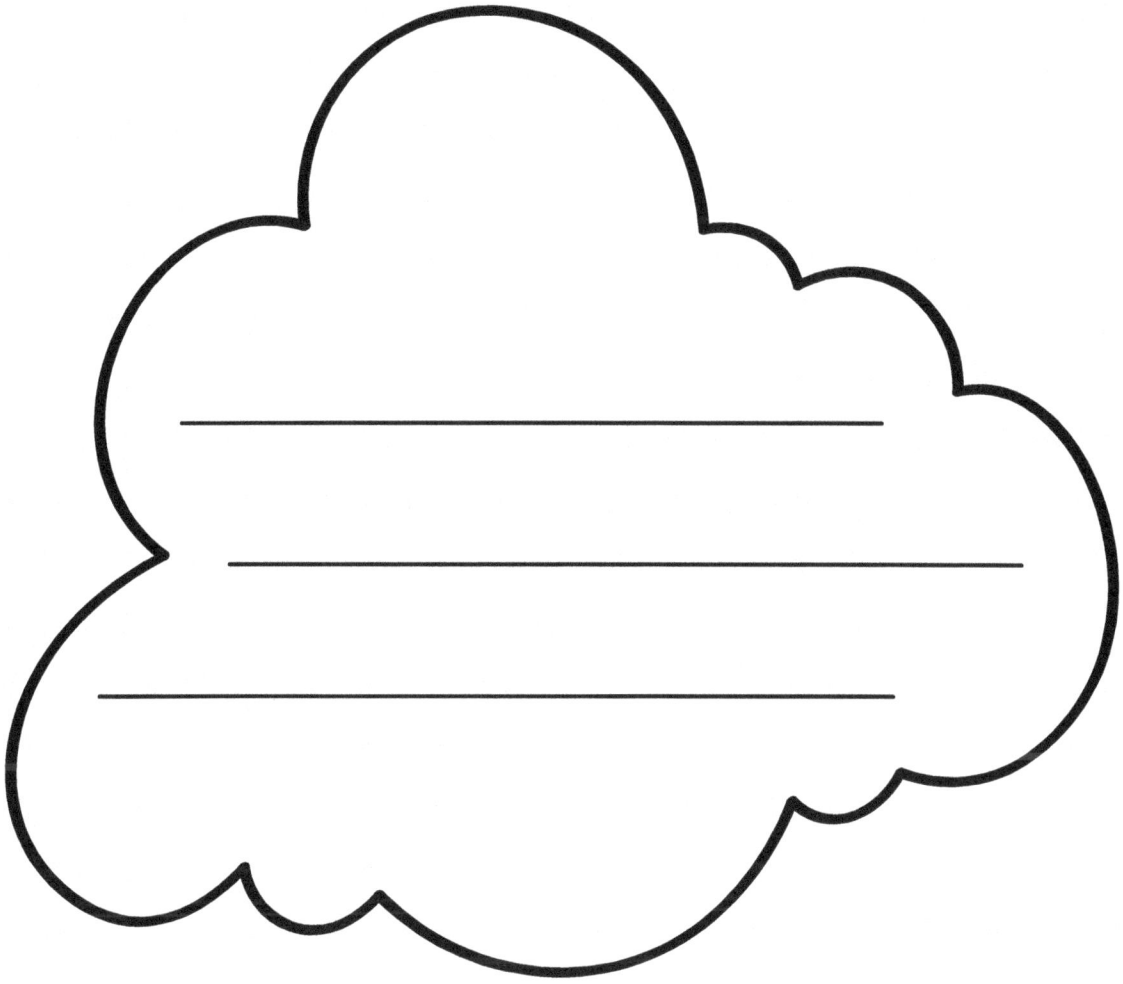

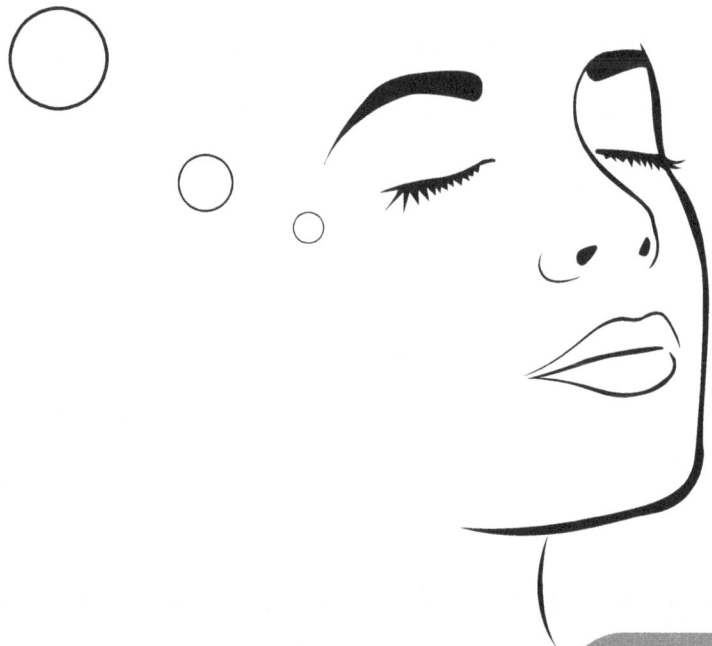

Reflective Practice

At the end of Day 11, take some time to reflect on your experience with affectionate self-talk. Write down any observations, such as:

- How did replacing self-criticism with loving self-talk make you feel?
- Did you notice any changes in your mood or self-perception?
- How did affirmations of self-worth impact your overall well-being?

DAY 12: Body Appreciation

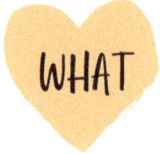

WHAT

Write down five things you appreciate about your body, focusing on its strength, resilience, and uniqueness. This exercise encourages a positive body image and helps you develop a deeper sense of gratitude for your physical self.

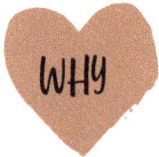

WHY

Body appreciation involves recognizing and valuing the unique qualities and abilities of your body. This practice helps promote a positive body image and self-acceptance.

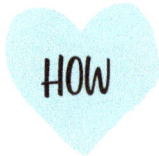

HOW

Practicing Body Appreciation:
- Reflect on your body's strength by considering physical activities, endurance, and any challenges your body has overcome.
- Acknowledge your body's resilience by considering times when your body has healed, adapted, or persevered through difficulties.
- Celebrate your body's uniqueness by considering its specific features, abilities, or characteristics.

SEE

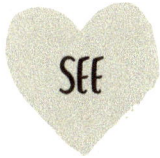

Examples of Body Appreciation:
- "I appreciate my strong arms that allow me to lift and carry heavy objects with ease."
- "I appreciate my resilient immune system that keeps me healthy and active."
- "I appreciate my unique eye color that makes me feel special."

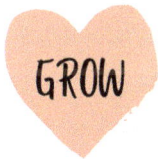

GROW

Incorporating Body Appreciation into Your Day.

Morning Routine:
Begin your day by reflecting on your body's strength, resilience, and uniqueness. Write down three things you appreciate about your body.

Throughout the Day:
Continue to practice gratitude for your body. When you notice any negative thoughts about your body, gently replace them with thoughts of appreciation.

Evening Routine:
End your day by reflecting on how practicing body appreciation impacted you. Write down any observations or feelings in your journal.

Note: *By incorporating body appreciation into your daily routine, you are fostering a more positive and grateful relationship with your body. Enjoy the uplifting and affirming effects of this practice!*

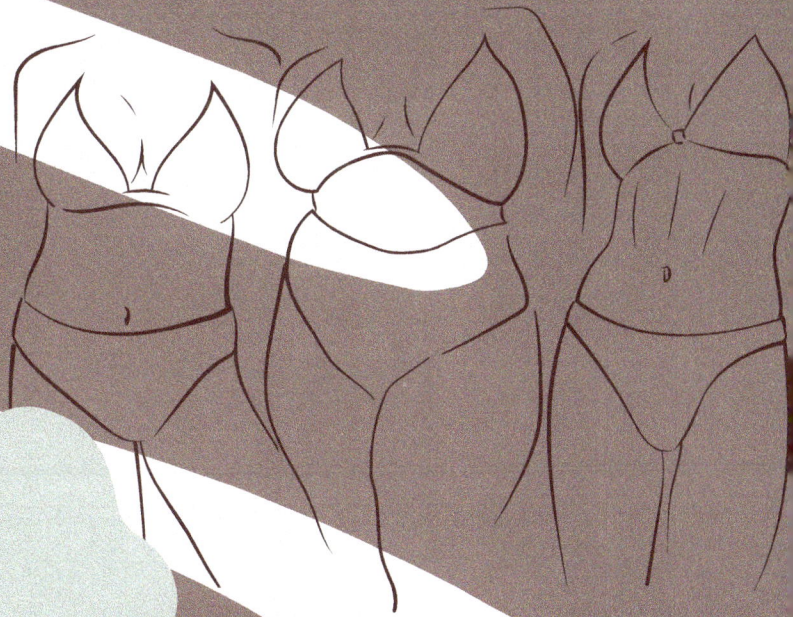

I Appreciate My....

Day 12

Reflective Practice

At the end of Day 12, take some time to reflect on your body appreciation exercise. Write down any observations, such as:

- How did focusing on your body's strengths, resilience, and uniqueness make you feel?
- Did you notice any changes in your body image or self-perception?
- How did expressing gratitude for your physical self impact your overall well-being?

DAY 13: Digital Detox

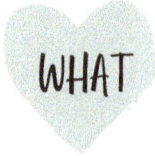

WHAT

Take a break from social media and digital devices to reduce stress and reconnect with yourself. Use this time to engage in activities that bring you joy and fulfillment.

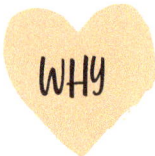

WHY

A digital detox involves taking a break from digital devices and social media to reduce stress, improve focus, and enhance overall well-being. It allows you to reconnect with yourself and the present moment.

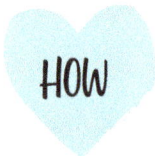

HOW

Performing Your Digital Detox:
- Plan how long your detox will last. It can be a few hours, a full day, or even an entire weekend.
- Turn off notifications and put your phone on airplane mode or in a different room to avoid temptations.
- Avoid using phones, computers, tablets, and other digital devices during your detox period.
- Plan activities that you enjoy and find fulfilling to replace screen time.

SEE

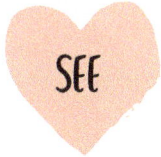

Examples of Screen-less Activities:
- Engage in creative activities such as painting, knitting, or playing a musical instrument
- Go for a walk, run, or practice yoga to connect with your body and mind
- Dive into a good book or explore topics that interest you
- Spend time outdoors, enjoying the fresh air and natural surroundings
- Connect with friends or family in person

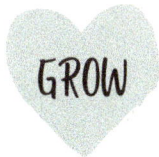

GROW

Incorporating Boundaries into Your Daily Digital Use.

While it may not be possible to fully disconnect in your daily life, there are still ways to establish boundaries. Whether carving out brief periods to unplug, silencing notifications to reduce screen time, or switching to airplane mode to stay focused on a single digital task, making these adjustments can benefit your well-being.

Note: *By incorporating digital detoxes into your routine, you are creating space to reconnect with yourself and the world around you. Enjoy the refreshing and revitalizing effects of this practice!*

Reflective Practice

At the end of Day 13, take some time to reflect on your digital detox experience. Write down any observations, such as:

- How did taking a break from digital devices make you feel?
- Did you notice any changes in your mood, focus, or overall well-being?
- What activities did you enjoy the most, and how did they impact your sense of connection with yourself?

DAY 14: Self-Love Playlist

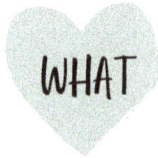

WHAT

Create a playlist of songs that uplift and inspire you. Use this playlist as a tool to boost your mood, increase positivity, and reinforce self-love.

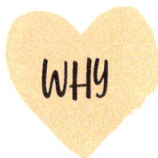

WHY

Music has the ability to influence your mood, energy levels, and overall sense of well-being. A well-curated playlist can serve as a source of inspiration and positivity.

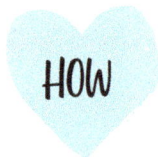

HOW

Creating Your Playlist:
- Think about songs that make you feel happy, confident, and motivated.
- Include songs that hold personal significance and remind you of positive memories or achievements.
- Mix different genres to keep your playlist diverse and engaging.
- Give your playlist a name that reflects its purpose.
- Listen to your playlist and see how each song makes you feel.
- Adjust the playlist as needed, adding or removing songs to ensure it consistently uplifts and inspires you.

SEE

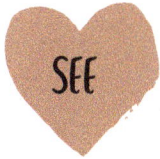

Example of a Short Playlist of Songs:

"Feel-Good Empowerment Playlist"
- "Happy" by Pharrell Williams
- "Stronger" by Kanye West
- "Unwritten" by Natasha Bedingfield
- "Fight Song" by Rachel Platten
- "Good as Hell" by Lizzo

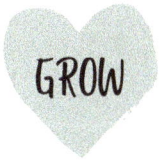

GROW

Incorporating Your Self-Love Playlist into Your Life.

Play your self-love playlist whenever you need a boost of positivity or during daily activities like exercising, commuting, or relaxing.

Note: *By incorporating a self-love playlist into your routine, you are using the power of music to uplift and inspire yourself. Enjoy the positive and energizing effects of this practice!*

Start Playlist

What song kicks off your playlist?

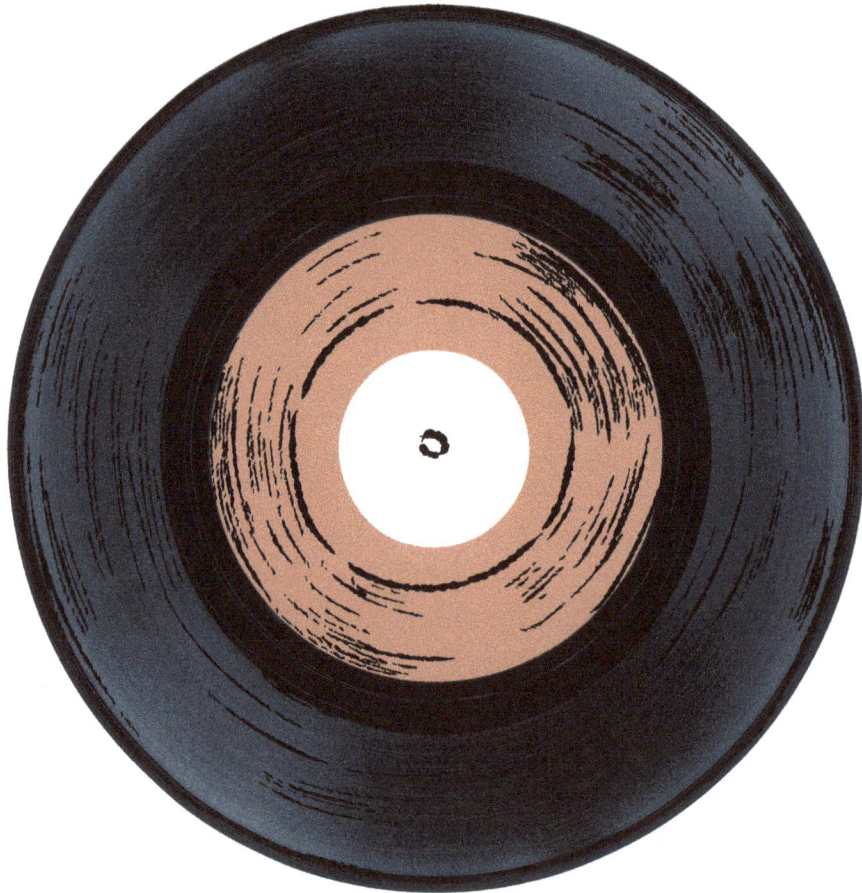

_____   _____
song title   artist

End Playlist

What song end your playlist?

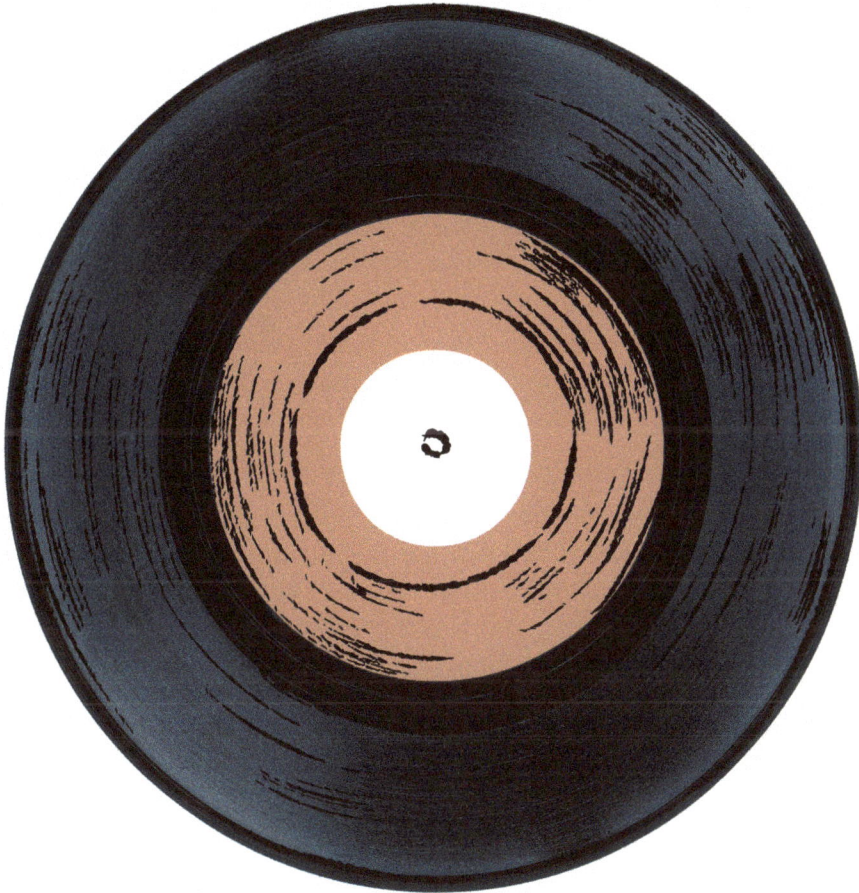

_____   _____
song title   **artist**

Reflective Practice

At the end of Day 14, take some time to reflect on your experience with your self-love playlist. Write down any observations, such as:

- How did creating and listening to your playlist make you feel?
- Did you notice any changes in your mood or energy levels?
- How did the songs you chose influence your sense of self-love and positivity?

DAY 15: Mirror Exercise

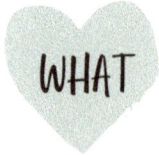

WHAT
Look into the mirror and affirm yourself with words of love and acceptance. Smile and embrace your reflection to foster a deeper sense of self-love and confidence.

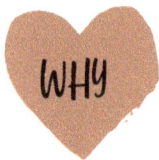

WHY
The mirror exercise involves looking at yourself in the mirror and speaking positive affirmations. This practice helps you build self-acceptance, self-love, and confidence by directly addressing your reflection.

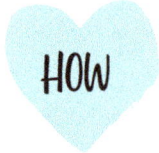

HOW
Establishing Effective Boundaries:
- Find a quiet, private space where you can stand or sit comfortably in front of a mirror without distractions.
- Think of affirmations that resonate with you and address areas where you need more self-love and acceptance.
- Stand or sit in front of the mirror and make eye contact with your reflection.
- Begin your affirmations. Say each one slowly and with conviction, truly believing in the words you speak.
- Repeat your affirmations several times, allowing the positive words to sink in.

Tip*: As you speak your affirmations, smile and show compassion to your reflection. Imagine you are speaking to a dear friend or loved one.

SEE

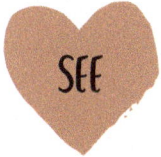

Examples of Affirmations:
- "I am worthy of love and respect."
- "I accept and embrace myself just as I am."
- "I am proud of who I am becoming."
- "I am beautiful, inside and out."
- "I am enough."

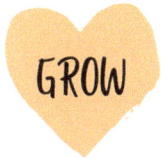

GROW

Incorporating Mirror Exercises into Your Day:

Morning Routine:
Start your day by standing in front of the mirror and speaking your affirmations.

Throughout the Day:
If you find yourself feeling stressed or down, take a short break and revisit the mirror. Repeat your affirmations to boost your mood and confidence.

Evening Routine:
End your day with the mirror exercise. Reflect on your achievements and affirm your worth and efforts.

Note: By incorporating the mirror exercise into your daily routine, you are actively fostering a positive and loving relationship with yourself. Enjoy the empowering and affirming effects of this practice!

Reflective Practice

At the end of Day 15, take some time to reflect on your mirror exercise experience. Write down any observations, such as:

- How did speaking affirmations to your reflection make you feel?
- Did you notice any changes in your mood, self-perception, or confidence?
- How did embracing your reflection impact your sense of self-love and acceptance?

DAY 16: Self-Discovery Assessment

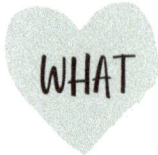

WHAT

Take a self-discovery assessment (personality quiz). Reflect on the results and what they reveal about you. This exercise helps you gain insight into your personality, preferences, and potential areas for growth.

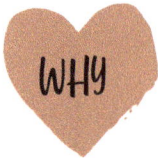

WHY

Self-discovery helps you understand your personality, strengths, weaknesses, and preferences. It can provide valuable insights into how you interact with the world and help guide your personal development.

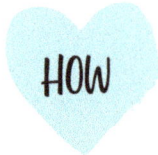

HOW

Taking an Assessment:
- Select a personality quiz or self-discovery assessment that interests you. There are many available online.
- Set aside some quiet time to complete the assessment. Answer the questions honestly to get the most accurate results.
- Review your results and reflect on what they reveal about you. Consider how these insights align with your self-perception and experiences.

SEE

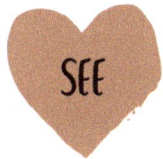

Examples of Free Online Assessments:
- Enneagram Test (*https://enneagramuniverse.com*)
- Big Five Personality Test (*https://bigfive-test.com/*)

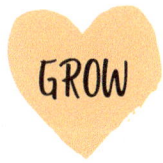

GROW

Planning for Personal Growth.

Use the insights from the assessment to identify areas for personal growth. Tomorrow, you'll develop actionable steps to address these areas.

Note: *By engaging in self-discovery, you gain valuable insights into your personality and potential areas for growth. Enjoy the process of learning more about yourself and using this knowledge to enhance your life!*

Reflective Practice

At the end of Day 16, take some time to reflect on your self-discovery quiz experience. Write down any observations, such as:

- How did taking the assessment make you feel?
- What did you learn about yourself?
- How can you apply these insights to your daily life and personal development?

DAY 17: Personal Growth Plan

WHAT
Identify an area for personal growth and create a plan with actionable steps to improve in this area over the next few weeks.

WHY
Acknowledging your room for growth allows you to focus on self-improvement and work towards achieving your personal development goals.

HOW
Creating Your Personal Growth Plan:
- Reflect on areas of your life where you would like to see improvement. This could be related to your career, relationships, health, hobbies, or personal habits.
- Define a clear and specific goal for your personal growth. Make sure it is measurable and achievable.
- Create a step-by-step plan to achieve your goal. Break down the process into manageable tasks that you can accomplish over the next few weeks.
- Establish a timeline for completing each step. Be realistic about how much time you can dedicate to your personal growth plan each week.
- Regularly review your progress and make adjustments to your plan as needed.

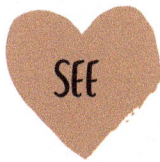

Example of a Personal Growth Plan:

Goal: Improve Physical Fitness by Running a 5K Race

Step 1: Research Training Programs
- **Timeline:** Week 1
- **Action:** Research and choose a beginner 5K training program that fits your schedule and fitness level.

Step 2: Start the Training Program
- **Timeline:** Week 2
- **Action:** Begin the training program, following the recommended schedule of running and rest days

Step 3: Join a Running Group
- **Timeline:** Week 3
- **Action:** Join a local running group or find a running buddy to stay motivated and accountable.

Step 4: Participate in a Practice Run
- **Timeline:** Week 4
- **Action:** Participate in a practice run to simulate race day and build confidence.

Step 5: Run the 5K Race
- **Timeline:** Week 5
- **Action:** Complete the 5K race and celebrate your achievement.

GROW

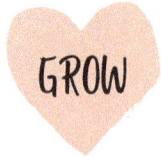

Incorporating Celebration into Your Personal Growth Plan.

Throughout your journey, take time to celebrate small victories. While reaching the end is the ultimate goal, recognizing your dedication and achievements along the way is equally important. Your commitment is what propels you forward, so remember to cheer yourself on at every milestone!

Note: *By creating and following a personal growth plan, you are taking proactive steps towards self-improvement and achieving your goals. Enjoy the sense of accomplishment and growth that comes with this practice!*

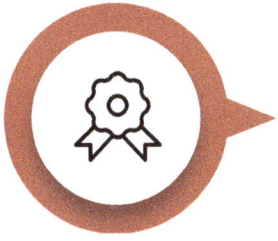

Set a goal

_____

_____

_____

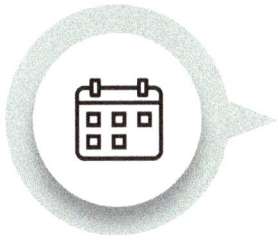

Set a deadline

_____

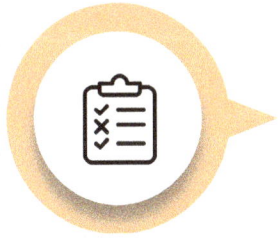

Create a plan

_____

_____

_____

_____

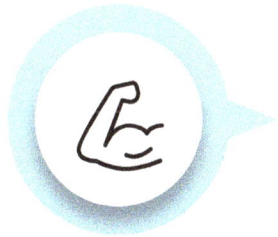

Take action

_____

_____

_____

Reflective Practice

At the end of Day 17, take some time to reflect on your personal growth plan. Write down any observations, such as:

- How did creating a personal growth plan make you feel?
- What challenges do you anticipate, and how will you address them?
- How will achieving this goal impact your overall well-being and personal development?

DAY 18: Nature Connection

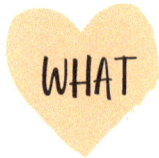

WHAT

Spend time in nature and reflect on the beauty around you, recognizing how it mirrors the beauty within you. This exercise helps you connect with the natural world and foster a sense of inner peace and self-appreciation.

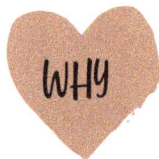

WHY

Spending time in nature has numerous benefits, including reducing stress, improving mood, and enhancing overall well-being. It provides a peaceful environment for self-reflection and mindfulness.

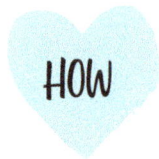

HOW

Connecting With Nature:
- Select a natural setting that you enjoy and can easily access. This could be a park, forest, beach, garden, or even your backyard.
- Set aside at least 30 minutes to an hour for your nature connection activity.
- As you spend time in nature, engage all your senses to fully experience your surroundings. Notice the sights, sounds, smells, and textures around you.
- Take a moment to reflect on the beauty around you and how it mirrors the beauty within you. Consider the qualities you admire in nature and how they relate to your own strengths and attributes.

SEE

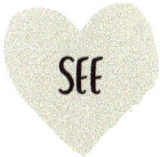

Examples of a Nature Connection Experience:

Location: Local Park

Sensory Engagement:
- **Sight:** Notice the morning sunlight filtering through the trees
- **Sound:** Listen to the birds chirping and the leaves rustling in the breeze
- **Smell:** Inhale the fresh scent of pine and earth

Reflection: "The flowing stream reminds me of my own ability to move forward, even through obstacles."

Gratitude:
- "I am grateful for the vibrant flowers and for my own creativity."
- "I am grateful for the sturdy trees and for my own resilience."

GROW

Connecting with Nature for Inner Peace and Self-Appreciation.

Spending time in nature fosters inner peace and self-appreciation, mirroring the beauty of the natural world within ourselves. It is essential to set aside time to engage with nature, allowing it to reduce stress, improve mood, and enhance overall well-being. Recognize the qualities in nature that resonate with your own strengths and attributes, and express gratitude for the tranquility it brings. By doing so, you cultivate a deeper appreciation for both the environment and yourself.

Note: *By incorporating nature connection into your routine, you are fostering a deeper appreciation for the natural world and for yourself. Enjoy the calming and uplifting effects of this practice!*

Nature Connection Prompt

Instructions: Set aside 30 minutes in a natural setting. Engage your senses as you walk or sit quietly. Record your observations on the spaces provided.

I touched...

I heard...

I smelled...

I felt...

I saw...

Reflective Practice

At the end of Day 18, take some time to reflect on your nature connection experience. Write down any observations, such as:

- How did spending time in nature make you feel?
- What natural elements did you find most beautiful, and how do they relate to your own qualities?
- How did connecting with nature impact your sense of inner peace and self-appreciation?

DAY 19: Creative Expression

WHAT

Engage in a creative activity that you enjoy, such as painting, writing, dancing, or any other form of creative expression. Use this as an outlet for self-expression and to nurture your inner artist.

WHY

Creative activities allow you to express your thoughts, feelings, and ideas in unique ways. They can be therapeutic, helping you to relax, de-stress, and connect with your inner self.

HOW

Expressing Yourself Creatively:
- Select a creative activity that you enjoy and feel comfortable with.
- Gather all the necessary materials and set up in a quiet, dedicated space to complete your activity.
- Start your chosen activity with an open mind and heart. Allow yourself to fully immerse yourself in the creative process without worrying about the outcome.
- After completing your creative activity, take a moment to reflect on how it made you feel.
- If you feel comfortable, share your creative work with others. This could be with friends, family, or a supportive online community. Sharing can enhance your sense of accomplishment and connection.

SEE

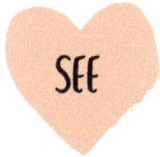

Examples of Creatively Expressive Activities:
- Painting or drawing
- Writing poetry or songs
- Dancing or choreographing a dance
- Playing an instrument
- Crafting or DIY projects
- Photography or videography

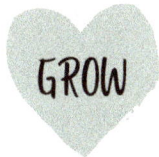

GROW

Embracing Creative Expression.

Creative expression is essential for personal growth and emotional well-being. By exploring various forms of creativity, you unlock your inner potential and gain deeper insights into yourself. This practice encourages innovation, reduces stress, and enhances your ability to communicate complex emotions. Embrace creative activities regularly to nurture your imagination and foster a sense of fulfillment and self-discovery.

Note: *By incorporating creative expression into your routine, you are nurturing your inner artist and finding new ways to connect with yourself. Enjoy the freedom and joy that comes with this practice!*

Reflective Practice

At the end of Day 19, take some time to reflect on your creative expression experience. Write down any observations, such as:

- How did engaging in a creative activity make you feel?
- What did you enjoy most about the creative process?
- How did this activity help you express your thoughts and emotions?

DAY 20: Support System Review

WHAT

Reflect on the people who support you and reach out to one of them to express gratitude for their presence in your life. This exercise helps you recognize the importance of your support system and strengthen your relationships.

WHY

A strong support system can provide emotional, mental, and sometimes physical support. Recognizing and appreciating these relationships can enhance your well-being and sense of connection.

HOW

Reflecting on Your Support System:
- Write down the names of the people who make up your support system. Note how they have supported you and what qualities you appreciate about them.
- Select one person from your list to reach out to today.
- Reach out and express your gratitude for their presence in your life. You can do this through a phone call, text message, email, or even a handwritten note.
- Take a moment to reflect on how it made you feel. Consider the impact it might have had on the person you reached out to as well.

SEE

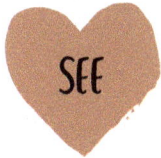

Example of a Handwritten Note of Gratitude:

"Dear Mom, I wanted to let you know how much your love and support mean to me. You have always been my rock, and I am so grateful for your wisdom and encouragement. Thank you for everything you do. Love, [Your Name]."

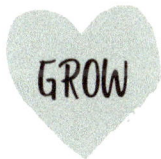

GROW

Reviewing Your Support System for Enhanced Well-Being

Be honest about the support you need in different areas of your life and take steps to cultivate meaningful connections. A robust support system is essential for navigating life's challenges and achieving personal growth.

Note: *By recognizing and appreciating your support system, you are strengthening your relationships and fostering a sense of gratitude and connection. Enjoy the positive feelings that come with this practice!*

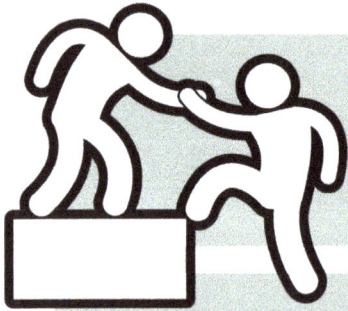

Strengthening My SUPPORT SYSTEM

Reflect on the strengths and weaknesses of your support system. Where do you feel most supported? Where do you feel gaps?

STRENGTHS

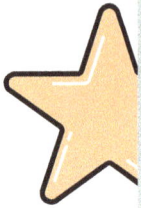

WEAKNESSES

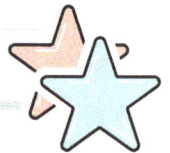

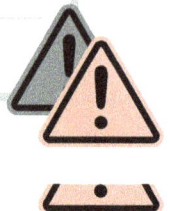

List specific actions you can take to
strengthen existing relationships and make new connections.

Set three goals to
enhance your support
system. Be specific and
include a timeline.

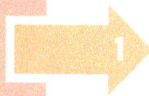

1

2

3

Schedule a monthly check-in to reflect on your progress. Record
any changes, improvements, or areas still needing attention.

DATE:

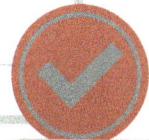

Reflective Practice

At the end of Day 20, take some time to reflect on your support system review experience. Write down any observations, such as:

- How did reflecting on your support system make you feel?
- What did you notice about the people who support you?
- How did expressing gratitude impact your sense of connection and well-being?

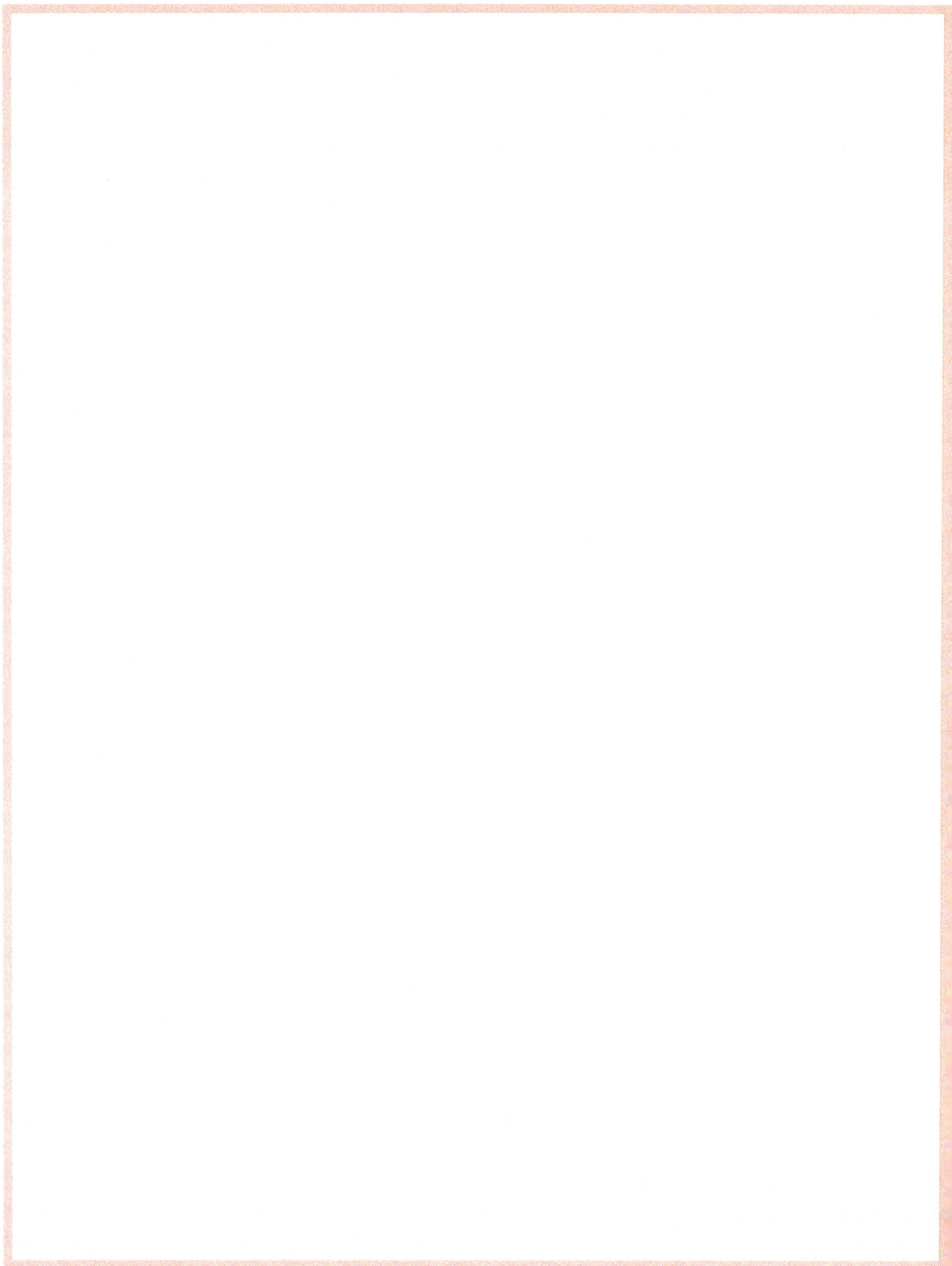

The Self-Love Challenge

DAYS 21-30 | REFLECTION AND INTEGRATION

Create

Vision Board

Practice mindful eating

Take a walk and reflect

Self-Care Day

Past Accomplishments

Self Reflection

Write your future self a Letter

Celebrate

Meditate

DAY 21: Self-Care Day

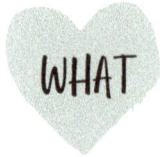

WHAT

Dedicate the entire day to self-care activities. Engage in activities that make you feel nourished, rejuvenated, and happy. This day is about prioritizing your well-being and taking time for yourself.

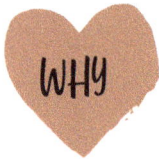

WHY

Self-care is essential for maintaining physical, mental, and emotional health. It helps you recharge, reduces stress, and improves your overall well-being.

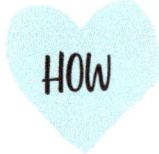

HOW

Preparing for Your Self-Care Day:
- Access your needs.
  - Plan to ensure you have a variety of self-care activities lined up. Consider activities that nourish your body, mind, and soul.
  - Set up a comfortable and relaxing environment at home. Clean and organize your space, light candles, play soothing music, and gather any materials you need for your self-care activities.
  - Reflect on what nurtures your inner self and brings you joy and peace. This could include spiritual practices, creative outlets, nature, and connections with loved ones.

SEE

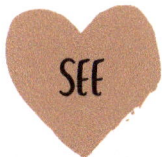

Examples of a Day of Self-Care:
- Engage in Physical Self-Care: Start your day with activities that take care of your physical well-being. This could include exercise, meal prep, and skincare routines.
- Engage in Mental and Emotional Self-Care: Spend time on activities that calm your mind and nourish your soul. This could include meditation, journaling, or spending time in nature.
- Engage in Creative and Relaxing Activities: Indulge in creative pursuits and activities that bring you joy and relaxation.
- End the Day with Relaxation: Wind down with relaxing activities that prepare you for a restful night's sleep.

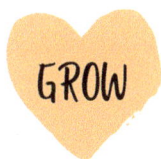

GROW

Prioritizing Self-Care for Enhanced Well-Being

Be intentional about setting aside time for activities that promote relaxation, joy, and self-reflection. This practice is essential for maintaining balance and resilience in your daily life.

Note: *By dedicating a full day to self-care, you prioritize your well-being and create a positive, nurturing environment for yourself. Enjoy the rejuvenation and peace that comes with this practice!*

Self-Care Day Plan

Objective: This worksheet is designed to help you intentionally plan a day dedicated to self-care, ensuring you prioritize activities that nurture your mental, physical, and emotional well-being.

This morning I will...	At midday I will...
In the afternoon I will...	This evening I will...

Self-Care Day
MENU

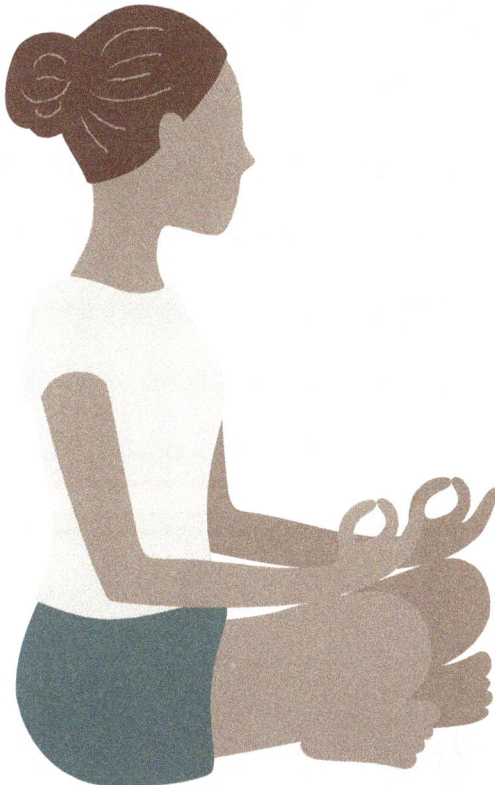

Starters

read

stretch

call a friend

go for a walk

listen to your playlist

Entrée

take a relaxing bath

learn a new skill

bake or cook

exercise

paint

Dessert

watch your favorite movie

enjoy a massage

do a facemask

have dessert

laugh

Day 21

Reflective Practice

At the end of Day 21, take some time to reflect on your self-care day. Write down any observations, such as:

- How did dedicating a day to self-care make you feel?
- What activities did you enjoy the most?
- How can you incorporate more self-care into your daily routine?

DAY 22: Reflective Walk

WHAT
Take a walk and reflect on your journey so far. Notice any changes in your mindset and emotions. This exercise encourages mindfulness and self-awareness, allowing you to appreciate your progress and identify areas for further growth.

WHY
Reflecting on your journey helps you recognize your progress, appreciate your achievements, and understand your emotional and mental growth. It also provides an opportunity to reset and refocus your goals.

HOW
Preparing for Your Walk:
- Choose a location where you feel comfortable and relaxed. It could be a park, a nature trail, a quiet neighborhood, or even your backyard.
- Dress comfortably and wear appropriate footwear. Bring along anything you might need, such as water, a hat, or sunscreen.
- As you walk, focus on your surroundings and take deep, calming breaths. Allow yourself to be present in the moment.
- During your walk, reflect on your journey over the past 22 days. Consider the progress you've made, the challenges you've faced, and the changes in your mindset and emotions.

SEE

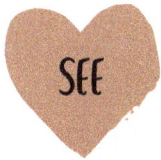

Examples of a Reflective Walk Experience:
- Example Preparation: "I'll walk in the local park. I'll wear my comfortable sneakers, bring a water bottle, and apply sunscreen."
- Example Reflection: "As I walked through the park, I listened to the birds singing and felt the warm sun on my face. I thought about how much calmer I've become since starting this journey."

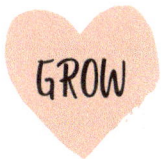

GROW

Embracing Reflective Walks for Personal Insight and Tranquility.

Incorporate reflective walks into your routine to nurture your mental and emotional well-being, gaining personal insight and achieving a sense of tranquility.

Note: *By taking a reflective walk, you create a space for mindfulness and self-awareness, allowing you to appreciate your journey and recognize your growth. Enjoy the peace and clarity that come with this practice!*

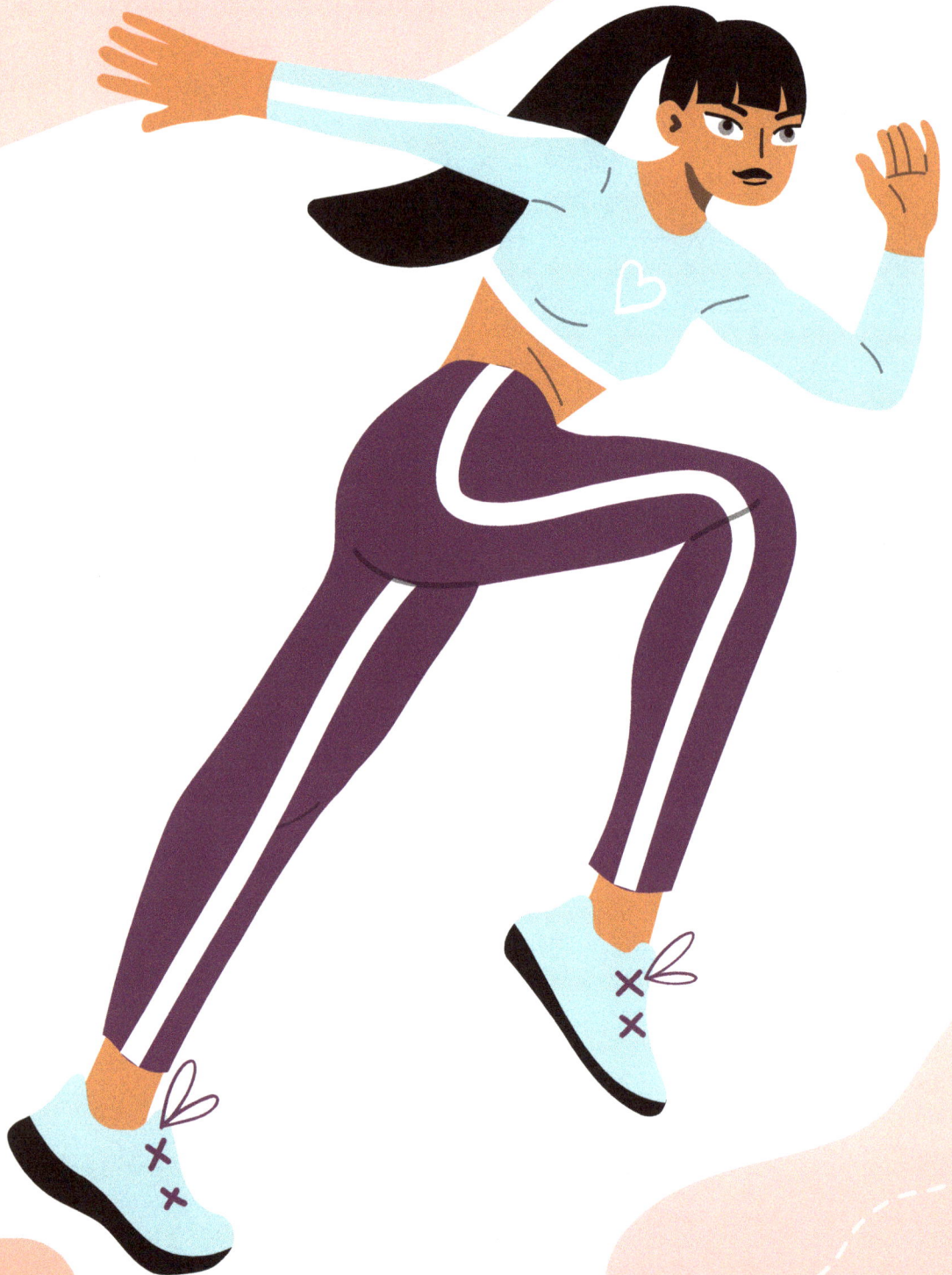

BENEFITS OF A
Reflective Walk

Day 22

INCREASE
ENERGY

BOOST YOUR
MENTAL
CLARITY

MAY
RELIEVE
DEPRESSION

IMPROVE
YOUR
MOOD

CLEAR
YOUR
MIND

Day 22

Reflective Practice

At the end of Day 22, take some time to reflect on your reflective walk experience. Write down any observations, such as:

- How did the walk make you feel?
- What positive changes have you noticed in your mindset and emotions?
- How can you continue to nurture these changes moving forward?

DAY 23: Vision Board

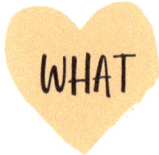

WHAT

Create a vision board representing your goals and dreams. Use it as a daily reminder of where you're heading. This activity helps you visualize your future, stay motivated, and keep your aspirations at the forefront of your mind.

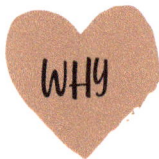

WHY

A vision board is a visual representation of your goals, dreams, and aspirations. It serves as a constant reminder of what you are working towards and helps keep you motivated and focused.

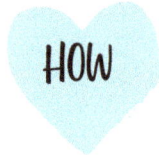

HOW

Creating Your Vision Board:
- Gather the materials you need to create your board. This can include a poster board, magazines, scissors, glue, etc.
- Reflect on your personal goals and dreams.
- Find inspirational images and words that resonate with you in newspapers, magazines, or online sources. Cut them out and set them aside.
- Assemble your board in a way that feels meaningful to you. Add any additional decorations to make it visually appealing.
- Place your vision board in a location where you will see it every day to keep your goals and dreams at the forefront of your mind.

SEE

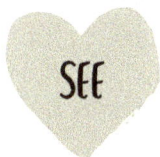

Example of a Vision Board Layout:
- Divide the board into sections for different areas of your life (e.g., top left for career, top right for personal growth).
- Place larger images in the center and smaller ones around the edges.
- Write or draw your inspirational quotes or affirmations.

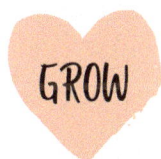

GROW

Incorporating Your Vision Board into Your Life.

Spend a few minutes each day looking at your vision board. Visualize yourself achieving the goals and dreams represented on the board. Allow the images and words to inspire and motivate you.

Note: *By creating a vision board, you visualize your future and stay focused on your goals and dreams. Enjoy the inspiration and motivation this practice brings to your daily life!*

Vision Board

ACTION PLAN

Personal Goals	Action Plan

Professional Goals	Action Plan

Health Goals	Action Plan

Financial Goals	Action Plan

Notes:

Day 23

Spiritual Goals	Action Plan

Relationship Goals	Action Plan

Travel Goals	Action Plan

Hobbies	Action Plan

Notes:

Reflective Practice

At the end of Day 23, take some time to reflect on your vision board creation experience. Write down any observations, such as:

- How did creating the vision board make you feel?
- What goals and dreams are most important to you right now?
- How will you use your vision board to stay motivated?

DAY 24: Mindful Eating

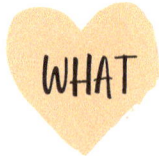

WHAT

Practice mindful eating today. Pay attention to the tastes, textures, and sensations of your food. This practice encourages greater awareness and appreciation of the eating experience.

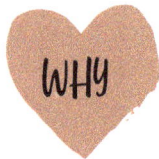

WHY

Mindful eating involves paying full attention to the experience of eating and drinking. It helps you enjoy your food more, recognize hunger and fullness cues, and develop a healthier relationship with food.

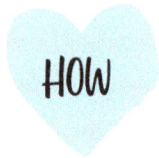

HOW

Practicing Mindful Eating:
- Set aside time to eat mindfully. Ensure you have at least 20-30 minutes to enjoy your meal without rushing.
- Create a calm and pleasant eating environment, free from distractions such as devices.
- Start your meal with a moment of gratitude. Reflect on the effort that went into growing, preparing, and serving the food.
- As you eat, pay attention to your food's colors, smells, textures, and flavors.

- Take small bites and chew slowly, fully experiencing each mouthful.
- Listen to your body's hunger and fullness signals. Stop eating when you feel satisfied, not overly full.

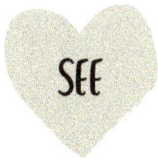

Examples of Mindful Eating:

SEE

Expressing Gratitude:
- Appreciate the farmers who grew the vegetables.
- Acknowledge the chef's work in preparing your meal.
- Cherish the abundance in your life that allows you to enjoy this food.

Engaging Your Senses:
- Notice the vibrant colors of your food.
- Savor the aroma of the freshly cooked meal.
- Feel the texture of the food as you chew, whether it's crunchy, smooth, or creamy.
- Taste the different flavors, whether sweet, salty, sour, or bitter.

Listening to Your Body:
- Tune into your body to determine if you're still hungry or full.
- Stop eating when you feel comfortably satisfied.

GROW

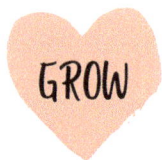

Incorporating Mindful Eating into Your Day:

Morning Routine:
Prepare a mindful breakfast and set your intentions for the day.

Throughout the Day:
Enjoy a mindful lunch and snacking, paying attention to the sensory experiences.

Evening Routine:
Have a mindful dinner and reflect on your experience.

Note: *By practicing mindful eating, you enhance your awareness and appreciation of the eating experience, leading to better digestion and a healthier relationship with food. Enjoy the newfound mindfulness and satisfaction this practice brings to your meals!*

4 Amazing Benefits of
Mindful Eating!

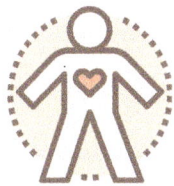

Feel better about yourself and your body.

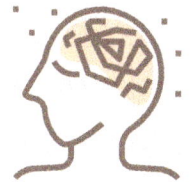

Reduce anxiety and depression symptoms.

Improve mood, energy level, and focus.

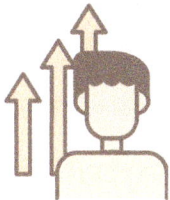

Help to manage your weight.

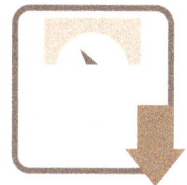

Reflective Practice

At the end of Day 24, take some time to reflect on your mindful eating experience. Write down any observations, such as:

- How did practicing mindful eating make you feel?
- Did you notice any changes in your eating habits or digestion?
- How can you incorporate mindful eating into your daily routine?

DAY 25: Past Successes

WHAT

Reflect on your past accomplishments. Write about how you achieved them and the qualities you displayed.

WHY

Reflection allows you to acknowledge your abilities, reinforce your strengths, and gain confidence from your achievements. It also provides insight into qualities and skills you can leverage in future endeavors.

HOW

Reflecting on Past Successes:
- Find a quiet and comfortable place without distractions.
- Think about your past accomplishments. These can be big or small, personal or professional. Consider different areas of your life.
- Write down each success and describe how you achieved it.
- Identify the qualities you exhibited during these accomplishments. Reflect on how they have helped you in other areas of life and how you can continue to use them.

SEE

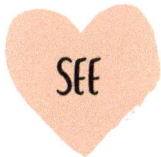

Example of a Reflection:
- "Today, I reflected on completing a marathon. I wrote about the months of training, the discipline I maintained, and the perseverance I displayed on race day."

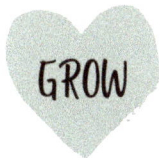

GROW

Celebrating Your Achievements

Give yourself credit for your achievements. Celebrate them and recognize the hard work you've invested, as this boosts your self-esteem, motivates further growth, reinforces positive behaviors, and ultimately fosters well-being and gratitude.

Note: *By reflecting on your past successes, you reinforce your strengths, build confidence, and gain valuable insights into the qualities that contribute to your success. Enjoy the sense of pride and motivation this practice brings to your journey!*

List Past Successes

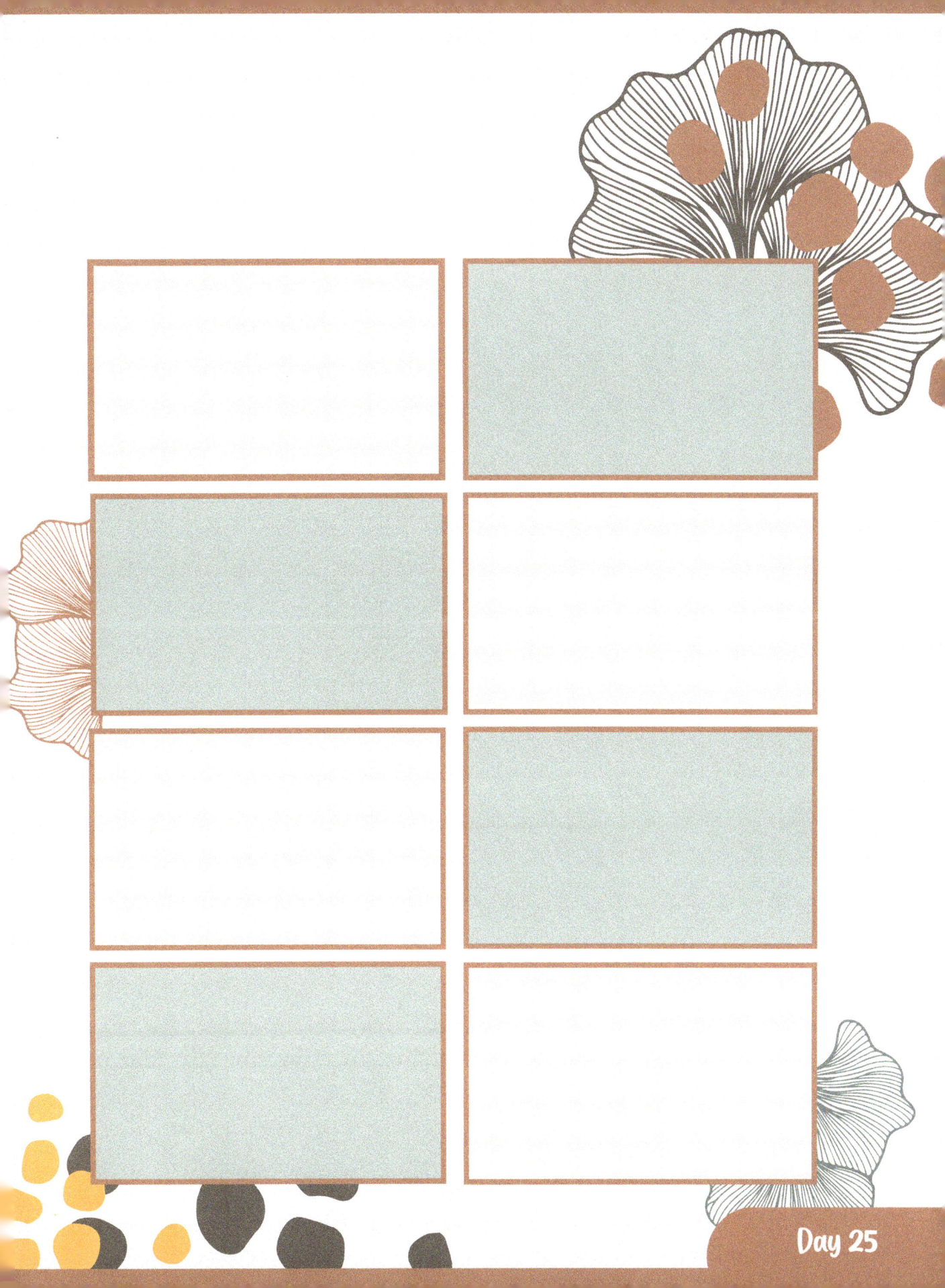

Reflective Practice

At the end of Day 25, take some time to reflect on your experience of acknowledging your past accomplishments. Write down any observations, such as:

- How did reflecting on your past accomplishments make you feel?
- What qualities do you recognize in yourself that you can leverage for future success?
- How can you use these reflections to build confidence and set new goals?

DAY 26: Future Self Letter

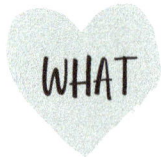

WHAT

Write a letter to your future self. Describe your hopes, dreams, and the person you want to become. This activity helps you set intentions, envision your future, and motivate yourself to achieve your goals.

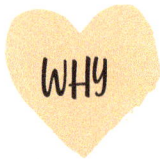

WHY

Writing a letter to your future self allows you to articulate your aspirations and create a vision for your future. It serves as a motivational tool and a way to remind yourself of your goals and dreams.

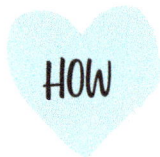

HOW

Writing to Your Future Self:
- Before you start writing, take some time to reflect on the person you want to become. Consider different areas of your life, such as personal growth, career, relationships, health, and hobbies.
- Begin your letter with a warm greeting to your future self.
- Describe your hopes and dreams in detail. Write out what you hope to achieve and why these goals are important to you.
- Describe the qualities and characteristics you want to embody.

- Offer words of encouragement to your future self. Remind yourself of your strengths and resilience to keep you motivated.
- End your letter with a positive and hopeful message. Sign off with love and anticipation for the future.

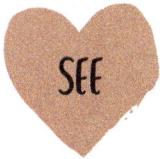

Example of a Handwritten Letter to Your Future Self:

"Dear Future Me, I hope this letter finds you well and happy. As I write this, I am filled with hope and excitement for what the future holds. I wanted to share my dreams and aspirations with you. I hope you have achieved your dream of becoming a published author. I know how passionate you are about writing and sharing your stories with the world. Remember how hard you worked on your first novel and the dedication you showed. I dream of living a healthy and active lifestyle. I hope you have maintained a regular exercise routine and continue to nourish your body with wholesome foods. Your health is so important to your overall well-being. I hope you are kind and compassionate, always showing empathy and understanding to others. Your ability to connect with people is one of your greatest strengths. No matter what challenges you face, remember that you are strong and capable. You have overcome so much...

already, and I know you can achieve anything you set your mind to. I am so excited to see where life takes you and all the amazing things you will accomplish. Remember to always believe in yourself and stay true to your dreams. With love and hope, [Your Name].

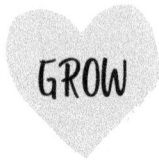

GROW

Incorporating Your Letter into Your Life:

Revisit your letter when you feel uninspired, letting it motivate you to keep working towards your goals. Extend compassion and encouragement towards your present self as generously as you would to your future self. Be kind and understanding during challenging moments, but keep moving forward.

Note: *By writing a letter to your future self, you set intentions, envision your future, and motivate yourself to work towards your goals. Enjoy the sense of hope and anticipation this practice brings to your journey!*

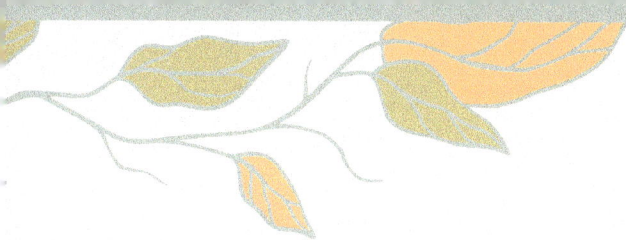
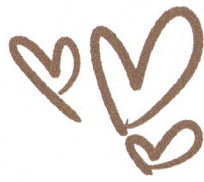
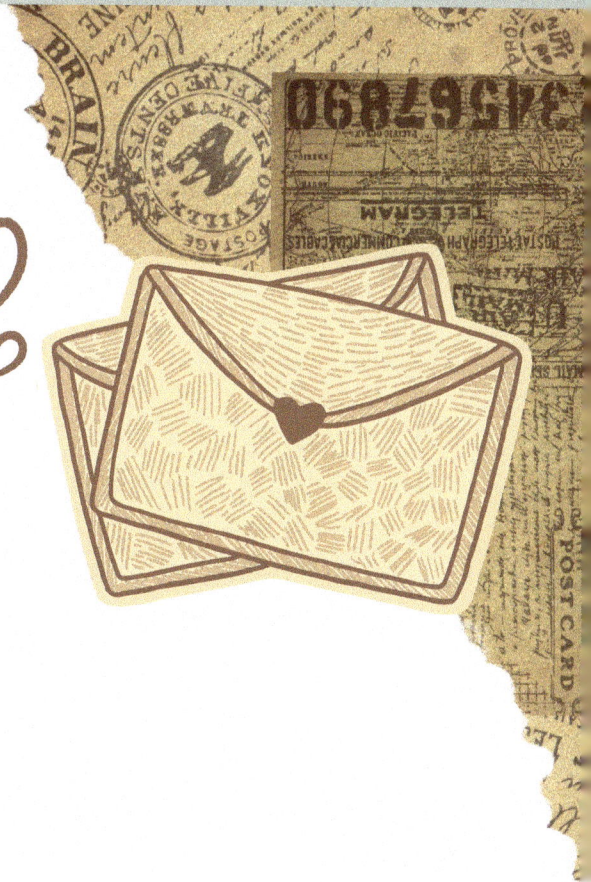
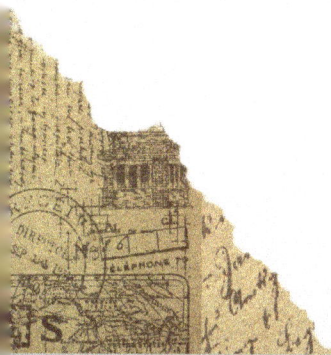
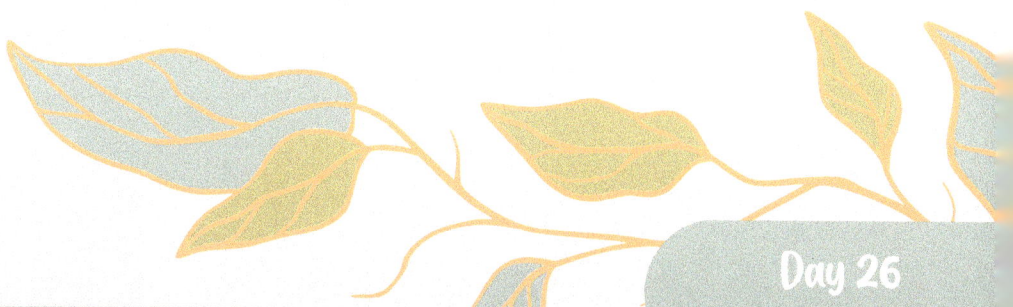

Day 26

Reflective Practice

At the end of Day 26, take some time to reflect on your experience of writing a letter to your future self. Write down any observations, such as:

- How did writing this letter make you feel?
- What insights did you gain about your hopes and dreams?
- How can you use this letter as a source of motivation and inspiration?

DAY 27: Meditation on Self-Love

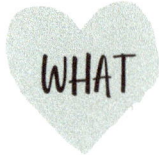

WHAT

Spend time in meditation focusing on self-love and acceptance. Visualize filling yourself with love. This practice helps you cultivate a deeper sense of self-compassion and inner peace.

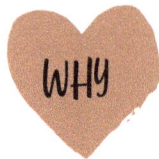

WHY

Meditation on self-love helps you connect with your inner self, fostering feelings of love, acceptance, and compassion. It allows you to release negative self-judgments and embrace your inherent worth.

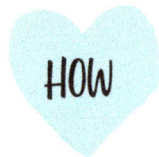

HOW

Preparing for Meditation:
- Find a quiet and comfortable place where you can meditate without distractions. This will help you focus and deepen your practice.
- Before you begin, set a clear intention for your meditation. This can be a simple affirmation or a statement of purpose.
- Start with a few minutes of deep breathing to calm your mind and body. Inhale deeply through your nose, hold for a few seconds, and exhale slowly through your mouth.
- Close your eyes and begin a guided visualization focusing on self-love. Imagine yourself in a peaceful and beautiful place where you feel completely safe and relaxed.

- As you continue to visualize, focus on embracing and accepting yourself fully. Let go of any self-criticism or doubt.
- When you feel ready to end your meditation, slowly bring your awareness back to your surroundings. Take a few deep breaths and gently open your eyes.
- After your meditation, take a few minutes to reflect on your experience. Write down any thoughts, feelings, or insights that arose during the meditation.

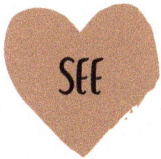

SEE

Examples of a Self-Love Meditation Session:
- Set the intention to cultivate deep self-love and acceptance. Spend five minutes on deep breathing exercises to calm your mind and body.
- Find a quiet spot in the park and visualize yourself in a serene garden. Imagine a warm light of love filling you and repeat affirmations of self-worth.

GROW

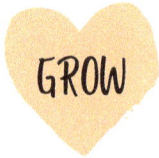

Cultivating Self-Love and Inner Peace.

Commit to cultivating self-love through focused meditation practices. Allow yourself to feel your thoughts and feelings without judgment to become more aware of negative thoughts and feelings that might prevent you from appreciating yourself.

Note: *By meditating on self-love, you cultivate a deeper sense of self-compassion and inner peace, enhancing your overall well-being and self-awareness. Enjoy the profound sense of love and acceptance this practice brings to your journey!*

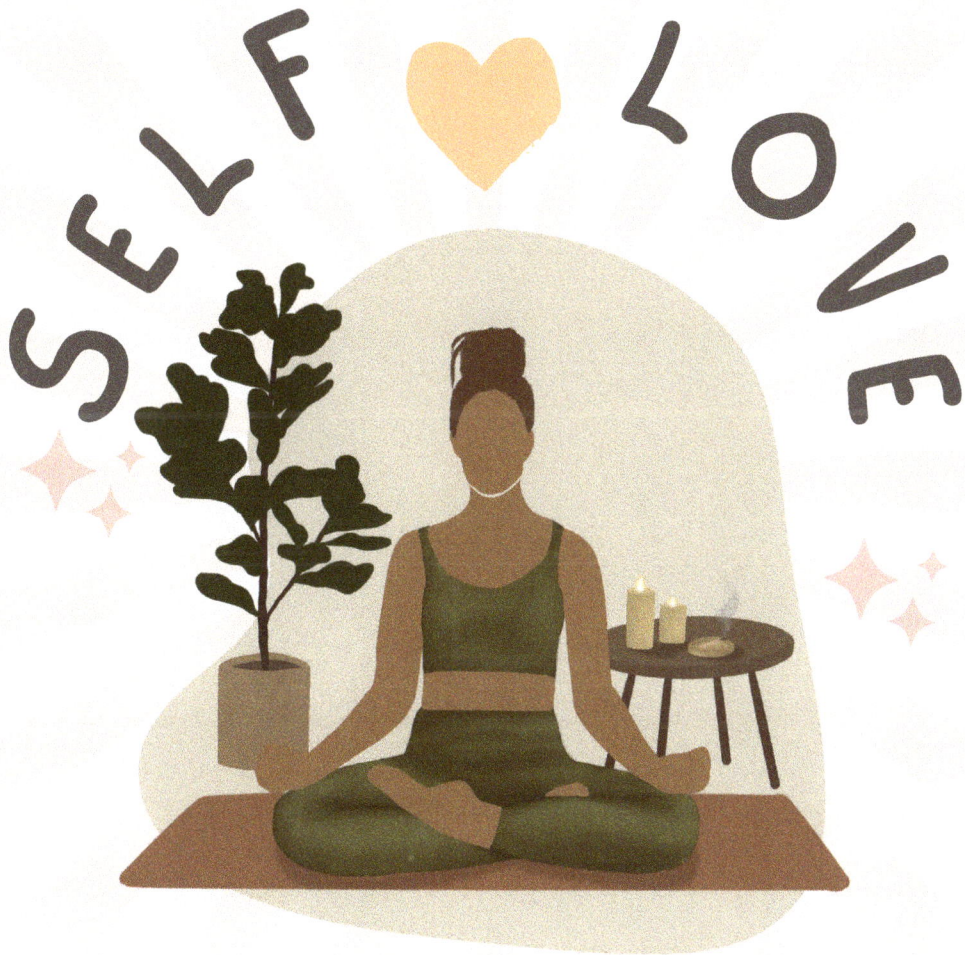

SELF ♥ LOVE

Day 27

Reflective Practice

At the end of Day 27, take some time to reflect on your experience of meditating on self-love. Write down any observations, such as:

- How did the meditation make you feel?
- What insights did you gain about self-love and acceptance?
- How can you use this meditation practice to foster self-compassion in your daily life?

DAY 28: Reflective Artwork

WHAT
Create a piece of artwork that represents your self-love journey. Reflect on the emotions and thoughts it brings up. This activity encourages creative expression and helps you visually explore and celebrate your self-love journey.

WHY
Creating artwork allows you to express your self-love journey visually and creatively. It can help you process emotions, reflect on your progress, and celebrate your achievements.

HOW
Creating Reflective Artwork:
- Collect the materials you'll need for your artwork. This could include paper, canvas, paints, colored pencils, markers, collage materials, or any other art supplies you enjoy using.
- Find a quiet and comfortable place where you can work on your artwork without distractions. This will help you focus and immerse yourself in the creative process.
- Take a few moments to reflect on your self-love journey. Consider the experiences, emotions, and insights you've gained over the past 27 days. Think about how you can represent these in your artwork.

- Begin working on your artwork. Let your creativity flow freely and don't worry about perfection. Focus on expressing your emotions and experiences.
- Reflect on your completed artwork. Consider the emotions and thoughts that arose during the creative process and how the final piece represents your self-love journey.
- If you feel comfortable, share your artwork with someone you trust or in a supportive community. Sharing can enhance your sense of accomplishment and provide additional insights.

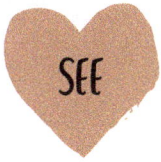

SEE

Example of Creating Reflective Artwork:
- Reflect on the key moments in your self-love journey, such as learning to set boundaries and practicing self-compassion.
- Paint a path winding through a vibrant landscape. The path represents your journey, with bright colors symbolizing moments of joy and darker shades for the challenges you faced.
- Share your artwork with someone and explain the meaning behind it. Celebrate your self-love journey.

GROW

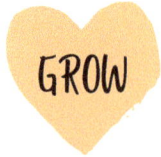

Creating Reflective Artwork for Personal Growth.

Engaging in reflective art can uncover hidden feelings and insights, leading to increased self-awareness, emotional release, and the development of a more authentic self. Additionally, the creation process encourages mindfulness and can serve as a therapeutic practice, promoting mental well-being and resilience.

Note: *By creating reflective artwork, you visually explore and celebrate your self-love journey, gaining deeper insights and a sense of accomplishment. Enjoy the creative expression and the powerful emotions it brings to your journey!*

My Artwork

Attach a photo of your artwork to this page.

Reflective Practice

At the end of Day 28, take some time to reflect on your experience of creating artwork. Write down any observations, such as:

- How did it feel to finish your creation?
- Who did you share your artwork with and what did you share with them about its meaning?

DAY 29: Self-Reflection Questions

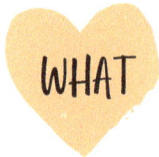

WHAT

Answer a set of self-reflection questions about your journey, challenges, and triumphs. This activity encourages deep introspection and helps you recognize and celebrate your growth over the past 28 days.

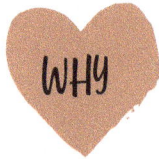

WHY

Self-reflection allows you to take stock of your journey, understand your experiences, and acknowledge your progress. It fosters self-awareness and provides insights into your personal growth.

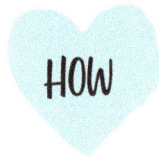

HOW

Preparing for self-reflection:
- Find a quiet and comfortable place where you can reflect without distractions. This will help you focus on your thoughts and feelings.
- Take your time to thoughtfully answer each question. Be honest and open., Allow your reflections to flow freely.
- Reflect on your responses. Notice any patterns, insights, or areas where you've grown significantly.
- Acknowledge the progress you've made.

SEE

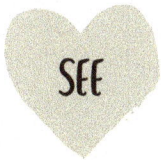

Example of How to Show Acknowledgement:
- Write a thank-you note to yourself, acknowledging your commitment to this journey and the positive changes you've experienced.

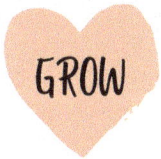

GROW

Engaging in deep introspection for personal growth.

Take the time to answer self-reflection questions to foster self-awareness and gain valuable insights into your journey, challenges, and triumphs. By engaging in deep introspection, you can recognize and celebrate your progress, enhancing your understanding of yourself and reinforcing positive changes in your life.

Note: *By answering self-reflection questions, you gain deeper insights into your self-love journey, recognize your achievements, and set the stage for continued personal growth. Enjoy the sense of fulfillment and clarity this practice brings to your journey!*

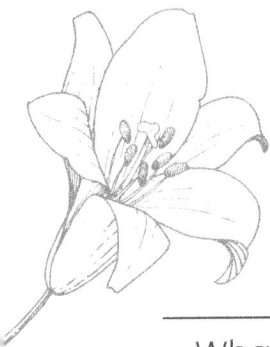

Reflective Practice

At the end of Day 29, take some time to reflect on your experience and answer these self-reflection questions.

What are the most significant changes you have noticed in yourself over the past 28 days?

What challenges did you face during this journey, and how did you overcome them?

Which self-care or mindfulness practices were most beneficial for you, and why?

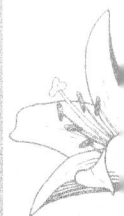

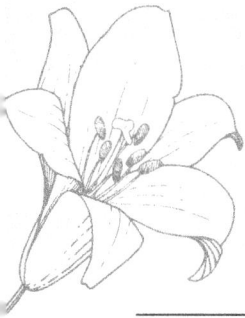
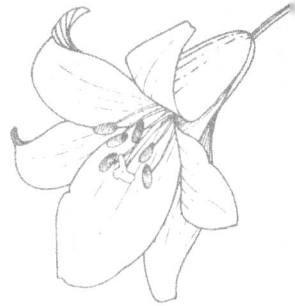

What moments or experiences during the past 28 days brought you the most joy or fulfillment?

How will you continue to incorporate self-love and self-care practices into your daily life moving forward?

Reflecting on your journey, what are you most proud of, and how will you celebrate your achievements?

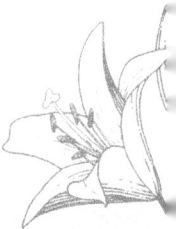

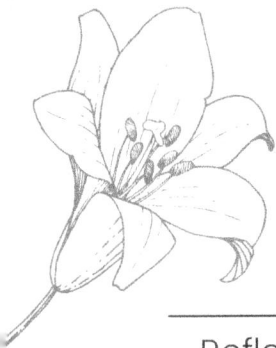

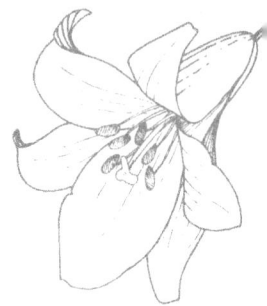

Reflect on a moment during this journey when you felt proud of yourself. What made it significant?

How have your perceptions of self-care and self-love changed over the past 28 days?

How do you feel about yourself now compared to when you first started this journey?

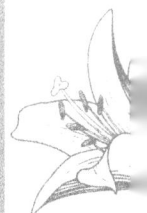

Day 29

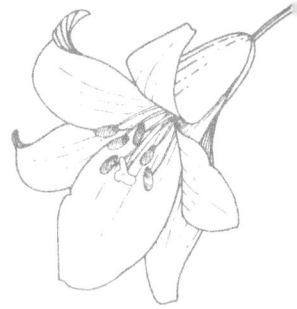

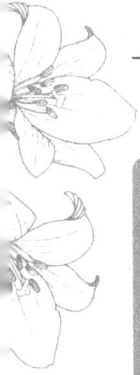

What advice would you give to someone starting their own self-love journey?

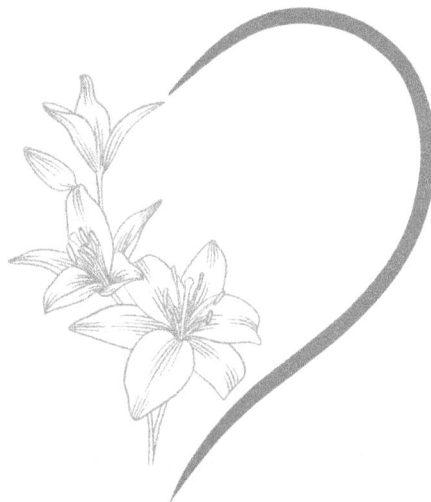

Reflective Practice

At the end of Day 29, take some time to reflect on your experience and answer these self-reflection questions. Write down any additional observations, such as:

- How did answering these questions make you feel?
- What insights did you gain about your self-love journey?
- How can you use these insights to continue growing and practicing self-love in the future?

DAY 30: Celebration & Continuation Planning

WHAT

Today marks the culmination of your 30-day self-love journey. Take a moment to celebrate your progress and achievements. Reflect on how far you've come and the positive changes you've experienced.

WHY

Celebrating your success reinforces the positive changes you've made and boosts your motivation to continue. Reflecting on your journey helps consolidate your learning and growth. Planning for the future ensures that the self-love practices you've developed become lasting habits, supporting your ongoing journey towards a happier, more fulfilled life.

HOW

Celebrating Your Achievement:
- Plan a special activity or treat to celebrate your achievement. Choose something that brings you joy and makes you feel appreciated.

SEE

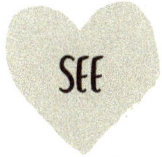

Examples of Ways to Celebrate:
- Spend time with a few people you care about and share your journey.
- Treat yourself to a nice dinner and a relaxing evening.
- Treat yourself to something sweet!

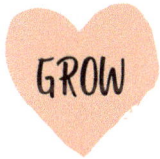

GROW

Celebrating Your Achievement and Creating a Continuation Plan:

Based on your reflections from Day 29, create a plan for continuing your self-love practices.
- Identify key activities or habits you want to maintain.
- Set realistic goals to maintain and deepen your self-love journey.

Note: *By celebrating and reflecting on your journey, you consolidate your learning, acknowledge your achievements, and set the stage for continued personal growth and self-love. Enjoy the sense of accomplishment and joy this final day brings to your journey!*

Reflective Practice

At the end of Day 30, take some time to reflect on your entire journey and the celebration. Write down any additional observations, such as:

- How does it feel to complete the 30-day self-love journey?
- What are the most valuable insights and practices you've gained?
- How will you continue to nurture and grow your self-love in the future?

Printed in the USA
CPSIA information can be obtained
at www.ICGtesting.com
CBHW041210170724
11734CB00024B/1525

9 798990 853263